Making the American Mouth

Critical Issues in Health and Medicine

Edited by Rima D. Apple, University of Wisconsin–Madison,
and Janet Golden, Rutgers University, Camden

Growing criticism of the U.S. health care system is coming from consumers, politicians, the media, activists, and health care professionals. Critical Issues in Health and Medicine is a collection of books that explores these contemporary dilemmas from a variety of perspectives, among them political, legal, historical, sociological, and comparative, and with attention to crucial dimensions such as race, gender, ethnicity, sexuality, and culture.

Making the American Mouth

Dentists and Public Health in the Twentieth Century

Alyssa Picard

Rutgers University Press

New Brunswick, New Jersey, and London

First paperback printing, 2013

Library of Congress Cataloging-in-Publication Data

Picard, Alyssa.
  Making the American mouth : dentists and public health in the twentieth century /
Alyssa Picard.
    p. ; cm. — (Critical issues in health and medicine)
  Includes bibliographical references and index.
  ISBN 978–0–8135–6161–5 (pbk : alk. paper)
  ISBN 978-0-8135–4535–6 (hardcover : alk. paper)
  1. Dental public health—United States—History—20th century.   2. Dentistry—United
States—History—20th century.   I. Title.   II. Series.
  [DNLM: 1. History of Dentistry—United States.   2. History, 20th Century—United
States.   3. Public Health Dentistry—history—United States.   4. Social Identification—
United States. WU 11 AA1 P5862m 2009]
  RK52.2.P53 2009
  362.19'7600973—dc22   2008035426

A British Cataloging-in-Publication record for this book is available from the British Library.

Visit our Web site: http://rutgerspress.rutgers.edu

Manufactured in the United States of America

"[O]rganized dentistry had no power to influence . . . underwriters and management, but when faced with the threat of a strike to enforce the same demands from unions, they acquiesced."

Joseph Yany Bloom, 1962

For GEO

Contents

Illustrations

Acknowledgments

A polymath community of friends and colleagues spread across several workplaces supported me in the writing of this book.

I had research help from the University of Michigan's talented and knowledgeable dental librarian, Patricia Anderson. At the Price-Pottenger Foundation in La Mesa, California, activist and archivist Marion Patricia Connolly set me loose in a gloriously (perhaps even perilously) freewheeling collection of documents. Research assistant Sarah Katherine Miller culled the files of the Wayne State University archives for news on the fluoridation debates in 1960s Detroit.

Teachers and writers Martin Pernick, Joel Howell, Regina Morantz-Sanchez, and Daniel Wilson, and University of Michigan Dental School dean Peter Polverini, each read this manuscript in early drafts; their wise comments enriched and encouraged this project. Historian Terrence McDonald looked puzzled at the idea, which improved it. Philosopher David Dick, sociologist Cedric de Leon, historians Karen Miller and Amy Hay, and the members of the University of Michigan American History Workshop contributed probing questions and enthusiasm. Periodontist Jill Bashutski produced the X-ray image of my mouth that appears on this book's cover. I am also grateful to Rutgers University Press editor Doreen Valentine, to copy editor Dorothy Meaney, to the Press's permissions manager, Christina Brianik, and to the Press's anonymous reader, for their direction and skillful work.

The image of the Kapaa School used in chapter 3 is with kind permission of the American Dental Association. The image of hygienists attending the National Dental Association's convention that is featured in chapter 6, and the Bioblend advertisement that appears in chapter 7, are used with kind permission of the National Dental Association. Materials in chapter 2 from the personal papers of Weston A. Price are used with kind permission of the Price-Pottenger Nutritional Foundation™, www.ppnf.org.

Financial support for this project came from Rackham Graduate School at the University of Michigan, the Regents Fellowship program of Michigan's College of Literature, Science, and the Arts, and the vacation provisions of the contract between the American Federation of Teachers' Michigan state affiliate and its staff union.

Staff, leaders, and activists at AFT Michigan and its locals gave me a window on the power and potential of American public schools, and on the strengths and weaknesses of the employment-based system of health insurance. Together with my fellow labor educators at Wayne State University, they also shared with me their understandings of the ideals underpinning some of the most memorable American programs of social reform. I am in debt to my colleagues in both places for their support of me, and of the big ideas that animate this book.

Ann Arbor
September 2008

Making the American Mouth

Introduction

I was sitting in a university dining hall one afternoon in 1999 when I found a curious advertisement in a copy of the *Wall Street Journal* that I'd scavenged from the building's recycling bin to read over lunch. In it, a Lexus logo floated in the middle of a small sea of blank newsprint. Above the logo was one line of type: "Naturally," it read, "all our children wear braces." Beneath it was another, the Lexus tagline: "The Relentless Pursuit of Perfection." The ad accomplished a lot with very little, and I was momentarily taken aback by how much its producers felt they could assume about *Wall Street Journal* readers.[1]

Where did the ad come from? How, in that time and in that place, did it seem so obvious that getting one's children's teeth fixed was "natural"? How could an ad seeking to trade on a shared stock of ideas for sales so comfortably assert that there was something normal, effortless, and socially sanctioned about the "relentless pursuit of perfection," and that such a pursuit ought to be carried out not only in automotive engineering, but in the intimate interstices of the human body? Why could the ad's creators be so certain that it was clear to every reader what counted as "perfection," anyway? There was no doubt, however, that the Lexus adwriter's finger was on a pulse that beat steadily and pervasively in American consumer culture at the end of the twentieth century. The ad's central assumptions about what *Journal* readers might consider "natural" were accurate, and this book is the story of how that came to be.

The Lexus ad, of course, was not the only place where late twentieth-century American consumers could find dental themes represented in advertising. Dentists themselves were aggressively marketing their orthodontic and tooth-whitening services in a wide range of popular forums, consistently linking the promise of healthy, good-looking teeth with the prospect of future success in all areas of life. A puff piece in a 1998 issue of *Town & Country* featured "smile designer" Larry Rosenthal describing his use of "ceramics, laser, and NASA technology," and counseling, "Think of it as a cosmetic smile lift."[2] Between 1996 and 2000, the membership of the American Academy of Cosmetic Dentistry doubled.[3] With relatively little explanation, popular news sources described the obsession with dental appearance as uniquely American: a *New York Times* article on tooth whitening quoted a London musician as saying "When I go on tour, I know which country I'm in because of the smiles in the audience. You know you're in America because of the piano teeth."[4]

Many of the foundational assumptions of the Lexus ad, like the surging popularity of aesthetic procedures and the reputation of late twentieth-century Americans as being possessed of uniquely good teeth themselves, would have surprised the dentists of the early twentieth century. These early dental professionals shared the Lexus ad writers' sense that good dental health could be properly read as a signal of other individual and national characteristics. But they despaired of convincing Americans, whom they regarded as having the worst teeth in the world, of the importance of good dental care. They would have been pleasantly surprised to find that their services had become such a "natural" adjunct to American class aspirations. They would have been shocked by the unevenness of Americans' access to dental care, however, and by the ways in which an income-linked disparity in access to services both reflected and contributed to increasing class stratification in the United States.

In the early twentieth century, Americans placed a low priority on dental health. Particularly among the working and lower-middle classes, it was common—and not considered particularly alarming—for tooth decay and gum disease to result in missing teeth. Because dental practitioners were comparatively few and surviving records of their work on individual patients virtually nonexistent, it is hard to quantify the prevalence of tooth loss. Military fitness examination records, however, provide some indication: in 1916 the army standard of dental health consisted of having "six serviceable double (bicuspid or molar) teeth," with at least two sets of opposing teeth on one side of the mouth and no less than one set on the other. One-third of all applicants failed this standard, and were rejected from military service as a result.[5]

The commonness of tooth decay and gum disease, and resultant tooth loss, meant that when early twentieth-century Americans thought about their teeth, they were usually thinking about pain. The misery of toothache itself paled in comparison to the iniquities visited upon a patient in the dental office, where he could expect to find dirt, blood, germs, an array of distressingly primitive instruments, and the occasional domestic animal. At the turn of the century, private dental offices typically lacked electricity and hot water; dentists used foot-treadle drills with slow mechanisms that made drilling more time consuming—and more painful. Ether anesthesia was available, but its side effects (most notably headache and vomiting) made it an unattractive option. Though the tenets of modern bacteriology were known to dentists, offices were rarely arranged in a way that made infection control possible. Private dentists' chairs were heavily padded with unsterilizable upholstery, and the business aspects of practice—writing out of bills and collection of payment—were often performed within feet of the dental chair. In 1907, a Russian exile dentist described the sanitary conditions of the New York dental office in which he found employment. "There was a distinct absence of disinfectory means," he wrote. "I can hardly express my feelings and surprise at seeing . . . absolute ignorance of asepsis and antisepsis. . . . My only answer, when calling attention to the above conditions, was a laugh from the dentist and his assistants."[6] Patients who lived in proximity to the few dental colleges of national renown could expect better sanitary conditions and more advanced anesthetics at college clinics, but they would typically receive care in large, open operatories where they were exposed to the agony of others' treatment, and vice versa.

Together with the sparse distribution of dental care providers, the unpleasantness of time in a dental chair made contact with dentists a rare event for most. The resultant historical memory of toothache in this era—epitomized by the image of a patient whose swollen jaw was bound up with a rag or bandana—correctly reflects Americans' propensity for self-care. Most people treated toothache at home with poultices, or with widely advertised patent nostrums—which, until the passage of the 1914 Harrison Act placing narcotics under the control of physician prescriptions, frequently contained enough opiates to make them very effective painkillers.[7]

Slowly, however, a variety of providers, of more or less reputable provenance, emerged to fill the unmet need for dental care. Legendary dental practitioner Edgar Randolph "Painless" Parker, who had obtained a DDS degree at the Philadelphia Dental College in the 1890s, grew a very successful business in the early decades of the century by exploiting both the shortage of other trained dentists and patients' fear of suffering. Parker invented and then popularized hydrocaine, a cocaine-based topical anesthetic, but his real appeal was aesthetic rather than anesthetic in nature. The practitioner, who traveled widely across the United States, cut a flamboyant figure in his jaunts around the country: he was well-known for his top hat and necklace made of 357 extracted teeth, all of which he claimed to have removed in one day. His entourage, which sometimes included a circus with acrobats, jugglers, tap dancers, and magicians, was specially formulated to appeal to working-class Americans, who had to take entertainment where they could get it.[8] Parker's brass band was particularly popular, though some speculated that it was provided partly to cover the noise made by Parker's own agonized dental patients.[9] This merry coterie of providers and performers helped Parker to collect millions in fees (at fifty cents per extraction) from patients who sought pain-free dentistry—or at least distraction—in the dental chairs of his traveling clinic. Later in his career, Parker established a national chain of low-cost dental clinics, which mirrored his exuberant self-presentation with alliterative signs describing the practices as "Philosophically Predisposed to Popular Prices." The Flatbush Avenue, Brooklyn clinic featured a block-wide sign reading "I am positively IT in painless dentistry," in which the word "IT" was almost two stories high.[10]

Despite his appeal to patients, Parker rapidly found himself in the bad auspices of the better-trained, less exuberant, and more reputable dentists of the increasingly prominent National Dental Association (NDA, renamed the American Dental Association in 1921), who regarded him as a charlatan and his conduct as a public health hazard. Partly because of Parker and others who aspired to his popularity, the NDA aggressively promoted laws and regulations restricting the practice of dentistry to licensed graduate dentists, and giving its affiliated dentists control over the licensure process. They described Parker as a "menace to the dignity of the profession." "Painless" Parker was arrested many times, most frequently for fraudulent advertising on the grounds that he was practicing under an assumed name, until in 1915 he legally changed his first name to "Painless," making it possible for him to use the moniker in his publicity without fear of prosecution.[11]

It was not uncommon for those squeezed out of dental practice by the new legislation and regulations promoted by the NDA to regard such measures as the hallmarks of dangerous collusion among a prosperous elite. "Painless" Parker, in his traveling lectures, frequently derided the NDA as a "trust" designed to ensure the maximum financial benefit for its members at the expense of dental patients. Parker's sense that the restrictive policies of the NDA were part of an apparatus devoted to the elimination of old-fashioned entrepreneurial competition was widely shared. The American naturalist writer Frank Norris, for one, regarded it as a fact so well-established that he could thread it insidiously throughout his 1899 portrayal of a self-taught California dentist, the eponymous McTeague. Like "Painless" Parker, McTeague was caught in the crossfire between self-trained craftsmen and better-educated advocates of a more regularized and scientific professional practice. McTeague prided himself on his status as a provider of a specialized service in a rough-and-tumble community, and on the increasing luxury of his office appointments, symbolized most vividly by the enormous gilded tooth his wife, Trina, purchased for display on McTeague's office signage. When served with notice that his early apprenticeship with "more or less of a charlatan" was insufficient to qualify him as a dentist under California's new state licensing laws (a letter that had to be read to him by his wife, owing to McTeague's illiteracy), McTeague stammered to Trina: "Ain't I a dentist? Ain't I a doctor? Look at my sign, and the gold tooth you gave me. Why, I've been practising nearly twelve years."[12] Thwarted in his business aims, McTeague later died in a showdown in the California desert, undone by the lack of a legitimate outlet for his festering, toxic greed.

In the early twentieth century, however, luxuries like McTeague's gold tooth were no longer sufficient to establish one's bona fides. The dentists of the largest national dental organization read them as signs of a suspect refusal to embrace the new standards of science and professionalism that were increasingly influencing American health care. Like the physicians of the American Medical Association, these dentists sought to incorporate the insights of the germ theory of disease, the refinement of aseptic surgical technique, the improvement of anesthesia, and new developments in bacteriology, chemistry, and materials science into their practices. They promoted preventative and reparative dentistry over the archaic standby, tooth extraction. Like their physician counterparts, dentists who had mastered these new concepts hoped to raise meaningful barriers to entrance into the practice of dentistry of those, like McTeague, who had not.[13]

Though they lagged behind physicians' programs of professionalization by more than a decade, efforts to standardize dental education and training in the United States roughly paralleled similar undertakings in medicine. Abraham Flexner's report on the state of American medical education, commissioned by the Carnegie Foundation for the Advancement of Teaching in 1910, helped buttress the case of reformers who advocated the closing of proprietary medical colleges and the standardization of medical training in the United States. As a result, the American Medical Association successfully advocated for the establishment of a four-year training period following two to four years of college as the standard for medical education.[14] In some respects, leading figures in early twentieth-century dentistry succeeded in advocating for similar change: from 1891 to the early 1920s, the training required of those seeking DDS degrees expanded from two years of practical training with no educational prerequisite to three years—often, at the best dental schools, with a prior year of college as a requirement.

However, debate within dentistry about how to standardize educational requirements for licensure prevented decisive movement in any one direction. There were three "reform" camps. "Stomatologists" argued for the establishment of dentistry as a medical specialty; advocates of the "level-technician" plan posited that lesser-trained assistants supervised by medically trained dentists should do most dental work; and proponents of the "reformed autonomous" plan advanced a more rigorous version of the existing standards for entry into the profession. As a result of this disarray among advocates of reform, dentists' educational requirements continued to trail behind those of physicians, and licensure to practice dentistry in most states did not require graduation from dental college. Many practitioners got their training through apprenticeships. Standards for the training of dentists and the practice of dentistry remained varied until well after the Carnegie Foundation's 1926 publication of William Gies's report on dental education, which helped to establish the "reformed autonomous" standard of a liberal arts degree followed by a period in professional school as the educational threshold for entering dental practice.

The persistence of a system of training through apprenticeship made entry into the profession particularly difficult for women, African Americans, and some recent immigrants to the United States. Prevailing cultural beliefs about the lack of mechanical aptitude—and low intellectual potential—of these groups meant that existing professional networks rarely expanded to accommodate them in apprenticeships. Formalizing educational attainment as the barrier to entry to the profession could make achievement of admission just as difficult. The educational institutions where training could be had systematically excluded female, black, and Jewish applicants, and without a network of amenable practitioners to depend upon, it was difficult for individuals from any of these groups to accumulate the professional endorsements needed for licensure.[15] The few women who were able to enter dental practice frequently confined their practices to the treatment of children. A similarly small number of African American dentists received training at historically black colleges. Despite their qualifications, they were often denied membership in state and local dental societies, particularly in the South. Because full membership in the National Dental Association, and later the American Dental Association, required joining one's local and state constituent groups, any dentist who was excluded from full membership in a state or local association was effectively excluded from the national group, though he was sometimes allowed the hopelessly misnamed "courtesy membership" at one or more levels of the organization. As a result of this segregation, black dentists formed their own associations at the local, state, and national levels.[16]

Debate within the profession about how—and how high—to raise the requirements of those who sought to practice dentistry insistently refused to acknowledge these omissions, focusing instead on the question of whether to erect barriers that divided white men (who, the Irish Catholic McTeague notwithstanding, were generally Protestant) from one another. For example, in 1926, the editor of the *Journal of the American Dental Association*, C. N. Johnson, described efforts to establish full medical training as the educational standard for dentists as the "pathetic apeing of those of supposed superior position in life," and proclaimed it "humiliating to the members of our profession who have any self respect."[17] In general, however, dentists regarded legislation and regulations restricting entry to their field as salutary signals of increasing professionalization in an occupation previously dominated by hacks. To these practitioners, adoption of the accoutrements of science and a resultant enjoyment of high social and economic status demonstrated a dentist's adherence to the emerging vision of "professionalism" in American dentistry. Recognition as professionals, they felt, would enable dentists to speak authoritatively to the public on matters of dental health and disease. This was, they believed, a task that demanded both advanced training and a sedate remove from the vagaries of commerce—something that "advertisers" like "Painless" Parker lacked.

The idea of professionalism enticed dentists in the early twentieth century, and debate over what would define the boundaries of professional status flourished even among those whom "Painless" Parker blithely dismissed as "the ethicals." Powerful voices militated not only in favor of qualifications like university training and state licensing, but for broader professional engagement facilitated by a proliferation of conferences and journals, and, implicitly, for the high levels of literacy and shared bourgeois norms of public interaction that facilitated such undertakings. Expectations for office behavior (of practitioners and patients) as described in major national journals hewed toward the gentility of the middle class. Both salaries and job security increased dramatically over this period, making dentistry a status pursuit on par with medicine and theology.

Together with the idea of professionalism, the question of what norms and practices would be defined as "American" interested early twentieth-century dentists greatly, and influenced their positions for and against certain kinds of interventions. Like American physicians, American dentists in the early 1900s participated consciously and overtly in an effort to distinguish American health care, including dental care, from that available elsewhere. In their view, a properly understood American version of health care would prioritize specific, expert knowledge exercised by master practitioners in clean, orderly, modern environments. The success of this sort of dental care was predicated on compliance from patients in matters of treatment and billing, but its providers also understood themselves to have affirmative professional and patriotic obligations to promote policies ensuring access to essential health care, including dental services, for the American public—and especially for children.

With very few exceptions, early twentieth-century American dentists were not socialists. Like physicians of the era, most were entrepreneurs who ran their own practices and felt strongly about their opportunities to command payment from patients, and to control the terms on which payment was rendered. Indeed, they frequently described these opportunities as the chief blessings of American citizenship. Therefore, like the architects of most contemporary American programs for social betterment—whether public or private—dentists aimed their activism not at leveling social conditions, but at "helping those who helped themselves."

Though dentists believed that government and private charities should avoid unnecessary largesse, which threatened to "pauperize" individuals who might be able to pay privately for their own care, they also believed that the existence of a large population of Americans with untreated dental problems reflected badly on their profession and on the nation as a whole. As a result, they often promoted measures that facilitated access to dental care in a hands-on fashion—particularly for children, but even, when needed, for poor adults.

By the end of the century, however, dentists had largely succeeded in their campaign for professional respect, and thereby had lost an important motivation for making dental care readily accessible to patients. Most dentists, and the organizations and publications of the dental profession, were firmly in the camp of individual responsibility for dental health care—adults, they thought, had an obligation to plan and pay for both their own dental care and that of their children. Dentists supported the fluoridation of public water supplies partly in defense of their professional prerogatives to make judgments in the area of dental public health. Yet they opposed dental insurance programs, and militated against the establishment and expansion of state and federal programs for the provision of free care to the impoverished. Instead, they promoted a new vision of dentistry as a method for lifestyle improvement, and a site for conspicuous consumption. Slowly, a consensus emerged—within and outside the profession—that Americans' teeth could be used reliably as an index of their personal or familial adherence to a set of aspirational norms about socioeconomic status and personal appearance.

As a result, by the end of the twentieth century, dentists increasingly defined as "American" government and professional policies that maximized individual providers' abilities to build and maintain economically successful practices, and promoted time-consuming, high-cost individual interventions to patients able to pay individually for such procedures. Orthodonture and tooth whitening could improve patients' appearances, gaining them access to the competitive, appearance-conscious upper socioeconomic strata. Even the experience of sitting in the dentist's chair was becoming the kind of indulgence previously enjoyed only by the very rich: in 2003, half of all dentists surveyed by the American Dental Association "said they offered some sort of spa or office amenity. Most common were neck rests, warm towels, and complimentary snacks and beverages. Five percent offered massages, facials, manicures and pedicures."[18]

Like physicians, dentists had once considered the promotion of such luxury crass. Propriety, they felt, required them to strive for the common good of the profession and the American people, rather than for narrow individual gains. They endorsed the subtle promotion of dental services that could be accomplished by a satisfied patient's display of her healthy, beautiful mouth. The direct solicitation of business, like that in which "Painless" Parker engaged, would never do: advertising both signaled a betrayal of one's professional peers and revealed that the advertising practitioner prioritized his financial gains over his patients' interests. During the course of the twentieth century, however, dentists' collective vision of how they ought to behave—as professionals and as citizens—slowly changed focus. The outcome was the conviction that both professionalism and Americanism required a system in which patients, practitioners and government held paramount the pursuit of the highest individual good.

The changes that took place within the dental profession during the twentieth century were, at times, hotly contested ones. The relatively elite group of dentists who controlled the major dental journals and professional organizations throughout the twentieth century were heavily invested in increasing the status of their profession, raising the standards of dental practice, and convincing patients of the importance of dental care. However, they faced opposition not only from figures like "Painless" Parker, who feared for their livelihoods, but from other licensed, reputable dentists who—while agreeing with the aims of reformers—disagreed with the specific methods the organization advocated for achieving them. After about the 1920s, for example, practitioners who were published in major national dental journals thought that annual tooth cleanings were essential, but dentists who read the journals and wrote letters to their editors, or responded to public talks given by advocates of dental hygiene, frequently disagreed. In the 1960s, professional journals urged dentists to become spokesmen for water fluoridation in their communities, but relatively few practitioners followed this advice, and some received it with open hostility. By the end of the century, authors and editors routinely genuflected toward the social and economic importance of orthodontics for those aspiring to the middle class, but dentists who served low-income populations—particularly those with large cohorts of minority patients—struggled to make basic preventative dental services available in their communities, and sometimes resented the feel-good message of upward progress articulated by the ADA.

Other workers in the dentists' office had to be persuaded of the necessity for change, too. The increasing presence of female dental assistants, hygienists, and lab technologists in dental offices reflected the growing specialization of dentists' work in the twentieth century, and meant that these auxiliaries' cooperation with new modes of practice (and of business) would be essential. In addition, other professionals needed to be deflected or rebutted when dentists proposed change that impinged upon their professional prerogatives: pediatricians, for instance, objected to dentists' claims that dentists ought to prescribe children's diets.

Finally, of course, patients had to adjust to the changes that a small group of comparatively high-status dentists sought to create. In the early decades of the twentieth century, though dentists increasingly prioritized "definite" and "orderly" systems of practice, patients continued to arrive late to appointments, object when they were asked to pay their bills "up front," engage in unseemly attempts to negotiate about fees, and question or reject dentists' judgments about what ought to be done to their teeth and when. Individual dentists—typically male, white, and Protestant—viewed these patient behaviors as annoying evidence of patients' gender, racial, or ethnic idiosyncrasies, focusing on the connections between patients' clothing, ethnic characteristics, and markers of social class, and their willingness to cooperate with treatment. For instance, dentists and hygienists who treated young children in publicly funded hygiene clinics in the nineteen-teens and -twenties frequently noted the hostility of "slovenly" and "superstitious" immigrant parents to the dentists' insistence that they stop feeding their young children coffee and garlic. Acceptance of such tenets, and alteration of a family's lifestyle habits, provided evidence that they had not only seen the wisdom of dental professionals' advice, but moved one step closer to successful assimilation.

The pace of the change that elite dentists sought in the twentieth century was significantly affected by patients' collective propensity to view dental health as important, dentists as admirable experts, and dental treatment as a necessary expense. Rejection of these ideas by early twentieth-century patients who were unconvinced of dentistry's value, and by patients who decided to defer or forgo needed dental care during hard economic times throughout the century, meant less business and less income for dentists. In turn, improvements in these areas helped to stoke the late-century increase in individualist cosmetic dental interventions. The *Wall Street Journal*'s 1999 Lexus ad spoke volumes about dentists' long-term success in convincing patients of these claims. Its writers could depend on the existence of a pool of customers (and aspiring customers) who had fully accepted the need for advanced dental care. The ad they produced on the basis of this assumption was a document rich with a language of mutual identification (addressing the reader as part of "our" group) and the sharing of common preoccupations (the "relentless pursuit of perfection" and the raising of children, for example).

At the end of the twentieth century, clothing, makeup, other bodily interventions like plastic surgery and exercise, and even the choice of leisure activities were sites for the communication of information about one's social standing.[19] Readers of the *Wall Street Journal* might have been expected not only to know this fact but to embrace it. The advertiser might easily have chosen to showcase instead the claims that "Naturally, all our wives have had breast implants" or even "Naturally, we all go to Cabo San Lucas on vacation." One of the things the Lexus ad assumed—through its reflexive deployment of this particular set of connections between cars and orthodontic care—was the existence of a shared stock of knowledge and beliefs about dentistry, in particular, among readers of the ad. Dentists' belief that adherence to dentists' advice was a sign of a patient's good judgment and social aspirations was reflected and reinforced by popular culture, as the promotion of "smile design" in the tony *Town & Country* magazine illustrated. That shared popular culture, of course, was intensely circumscribed by boundaries of class, race, and gender: it's revealing not only that the Lexus ad appeared at all, but where it appeared, and who might have been expected to read and respond to it.

Whatever the Lexus ad writers might have thought, there was nothing historically obvious or inevitable, and still less "natural," about the understanding of the role of orthodontic care for children in creating and demonstrating socioeconomic status that was displayed in their work. Though social pressure provided powerful impetus for Americans' participation in an increasingly costly culture of personal aesthetic improvement, dentists' vigorous efforts to assert their own professional interests played the largest role in bringing the new model of individualistic intervention to fruition. You couldn't have proven this by my own adolescent experiences, however: I had eight years of orthodonture in a suburb of New Jersey where we teenagers could identify one another's social status not only by clothing, parents' occupation, and location of our homes in old or new developments, but also by which of the two orthodontists in town our parents had chosen to fix our teeth. (My orthodontist, by virtue of having a second office located in nearby Princeton, was considered the ritzier of the two.) These providers advertised their services minimally, if at all. It would have surprised most of us, and our parents, to hear that they and their professional organizations—and particularly the ADA—had played such an active role in shaping our shared belief that it was important to have straight teeth. Nevertheless, reflection on popular-culture manifestations of Americans' thinking about dentistry can help to illuminate not only the moments at which dentists' ideas about teeth and their care were adopted and by whom, but also the moments at which those ideas were contested, and how that contestation contributed to the stock of American notions about dentistry and its importance.

Ten years ago, as I chatted at a party with an acquaintance who had grown up poor in Ireland, he remarked wryly about "you Americans and your teeth!" I knew right away what he was talking about—those eight years of visits to the orthodontist's office were vivid in my mind—but I had not thought about the ways in which inquiring into my own experience of dental care as a marker of class, education, nation, and age might provide the basis for an engaging or useful historical project. In this book, I try to demonstrate how the connections I lived at the end of the twentieth century were formed, while tracing the ways in which dentists used the opportunity to make and re-make such linkages in order to build their self-images (and the lay public's image of them) as health care professionals. This book has things in common with other histories of medicine and public health, and of the development of the health professions, but it also seeks to engage with histories of consumer culture and behavior, and with work that explores the ways in which American identities have been shaped and re-shaped in the twentieth century. It offers a new view of how these diverse bodies of literature connect, and a history of the ideas that grew where these streams of American life came together.

Chapter 1

American Dental Hygiene

"Small Flags Attached to Toothbrushes May Be Waved"

In 1910, the eyes of dentists around the country fixed on Cleveland, Ohio, and its suburbs. There, local officials, in cooperation with the Oral Hygiene Committee of the National Dental Association, had begun a new program of publicly funded oral hygiene education and dental prophylaxis for schoolchildren. Dentists hoped that the program would help to persuade Americans of the importance of preventative dental care and periodic consultation with licensed dentists to overall good health. The results of this program would profoundly shape Americans' ideas about what could and ought to be done for children's dental health, as well as their ideas about what habits of oral hygiene and health could be properly regarded as American. School oral hygiene programs helped link national identity with good dental health and an aesthetically pleasing appearance. Simultaneously, these programs influenced contemporary ideas about the roles of the school and the state, the constructions of childhood and citizenship, and the gender roles of dental health care workers.

Cleveland, Ohio, offered several advantages to dentists hoping to demonstrate the value of a publicly supported oral hygiene campaign. It was a thriving manufacturing city and an attractive place of landing for immigrant workers, whom dentists regarded as particularly in need of dental care because of their low incomes, poor health, and intransigent refusal to adapt to American ways of life. Among Cleveland's immigrants were significant numbers of Jews and Italians. Dentists, like turn-of-the-century social workers, regarded these two groups as the most difficult to assimilate; if the hygiene program worked in Cleveland, it could work anywhere. Cleveland had large and active state and local dental societies whose members were willing to participate in an oral hygiene campaign. The city was the home of several nationally prominent dentists who held powerful positions in the increasingly visible National Dental Association. Most importantly, the local school board and government officials were cooperative. National dental leaders trusted them to participate in the program without playing favorites or indulging in the practices of corrupt government (like taking bribes or seeking kickbacks) so common among early twentieth-century politicians, and so feared by scientifically minded bureaucrats everywhere.

Local planners expected the inauguration of the Cleveland campaign to be an event of national significance. The President of the United States, William Howard Taft, and the governors of all the states were invited to attend the March 1910 kickoff, which lasted for an entire afternoon and evening and featured speeches by local, state, and national figures in politics and dentistry, as well as musical performances by several groups of Cleveland schoolchildren. Though Taft himself did not attend, he sent a former assistant surgeon general as his personal representative. *The Dental Brief*, one of several prominent national professional journals, carried the entire proceedings of the opening rally in its May, June, and July issues, and referred to the campaign as "the greatest ever organized for the abolition of disease."[1]

There were several components to the program begun in Cleveland that winter. Fifty-six thousand primary school students were to have their mouths examined ("by a dentist and a lady assistant"),[2] with reports on their dental health to be sent to their parents, and free dental service was to be provided to those whose parents indicated that they could not afford to pay for reparative work. To serve the latter purpose, four school-based clinics would be established, and transportation provided to children from non-clinic elementary schools. "Best of all, if there is a best," announced the superintendent of Cleveland public schools, "is the lecture program, which proposes to place before young and old the preventatives for many of the troubles which are to be treated by this inspection and clinical service."[3]

Cleveland dentists and school officials explicitly linked the new oral hygiene program with their aspirations of inculcating good citizenship in their youthful charges. "The children of to-day—the citizens of tomorrow," rhapsodized the president of the Cleveland Board of Education, "by health, vigor, and education, well balanced, will the preservation of all the civilization and virtues, for which this government stands in the eye of the world to-day, be most surely conserved."[4] Several speakers commented on the direct links between health, happiness, and domestic tranquility: the assistant superintendent of schools even extended an oft-repeated dentists' phrase about the importance of good teeth to good health, arguing that good teeth were a preventative against bad politics. "Without good sound teeth no mastication, without mastication no complete digestion, without digestion no thorough assimilation, without assimilation what becomes of disposition? It becomes degraded, it becomes harsh and sour, and the end thereof is not sound government, is not nobility of life and character, but the end thereof is anarchy, and all those things that men who do not feel good within themselves, are trying to put upon the world without."[5]

There seemed to be no better place to test this latter proposition than in the Marion Elementary School, "in the Ghetto of Cleveland"[6] as one dental journal put it, where bad dental health had plagued a group of almost nine hundred students and their teachers for as long as anyone could remember. "All of its pupils are the children of people in very moderate circumstances," one editor reported. "Many of them are the children of wretchedly poor parents. A large proportion of the children are of Hebraic extraction."[7] Because Jews and the poor were widely believed to be prone to political radicalism and other kinds of bad citizenship, the Marion School population was especially attractive to dentists who wanted to conduct a special study, a subset of the larger Cleveland project, to determine exactly how much of an influence bad teeth had on pupil behavior. After preliminary inspection of the teeth of all the students in the school, dentists selected the forty students with the worst dental health for inclusion in a group known as the Marion School Dental Class (or Dental Squad). They offered these children free dental care and a five-dollar gold piece, which students would receive on Christmas, if they cooperated with all of their dentists' and teachers' directions, submitted to complete dental treatment, and performed all the tasks required of them "with proper spirit."[8]

The results of the study were eye-opening. Twenty-eight students continued in the study long enough to be evaluated for their progress in December of 1910: by the account of the Marion School dentist, their health and dispositions improved dramatically in the interim. Children who had been "ill-kept . . . sallow . . . [with a general look of neglect]" became "clean, bright, and healthy, with clearer complexions."[9] Extensive psychological testing of the children revealed that their average intellectual improvement (as measured by "increase in working efficiency") was 54 percent: some students showed gains even more astounding, of up to 426.9 percent as determined by tests of memory, spontaneous association, addition, and "quickness and accuracy of perception."[10] Most importantly, however, was the dramatic improvement in the pupils' classroom behavior: "A spirit of self-respect was engendered that corrected disobedience, truancy, and incorrigibility," the Marion School principal reported.[11] In her opinion, these students' new self-respect and better attitudes made them better prepared for citizenship: "I cannot too strongly recommend a prominent place to oral hygiene for all of us who are trying to conserve the child physically, mentally, morally and fit him for his place as a citizen of the United States."[12]

A five-dollar gold piece would have been a formidable sum to a child in 1910, comparable to what was then perceived as the most generous weekly salary available to a workingman, and a substantial incentive to participation in the study. However, the Marion School dentist and dental hygienist took great pride in reporting that, at the conclusion of the study, the pupils participating in it had "continued just as faithfully ever since": that is, that they had fully internalized the "gospel" of dental hygiene, and had in many cases gone on to propagate that gospel in their own homes. Though the children's parents, in the opinion of the school dentists, had originally been "with the exception of two or three, too ignorant to appreciate the value of the work being done for their children," at the end of the study some of them were following programs of oral hygiene too. In one family, "the mother is so delighted with results in the child that she follows my instructions in mastication, etc., and is improved," reported the dental hygienist.[13] One student relayed that her "father and mother thank you most heartily for the efforts and devotions shown towards me."[14] The Marion School program seemed to be making not just children, but also their parents, more perceptive and more grateful for the ministrations of professionals. This was one of the fondest hopes of the studies' planners, who regarded children as the gateways to immigrant households, and were optimistic about the prospect of changing the behavior of all family members by improving children's behavior first.

The Marion School Squad catapulted to fame in the world of professional dentistry. Dentists and scientists from around the country visited the school to witness the newly improved dental health and personal behavior of the students. A wide range of journals reported on the amazing results of their efforts, and in May of 1911 the *Cleveland Press* announced that the twenty-eight children were scheduled to appear in person before the annual meeting of the National Dental Association, "to show the results of the year's experiment."[15] Several journals published statements from the students themselves, and the *Dental Digest* ran essays by Marion School students Lillian Gottfried, Ben Dimendstein, and Lillian Cohen, reflecting on their experiences and on the importance of healthy teeth. "My parents have never believed that an unhealthy mouth would make an unhealthy child," Lillian Gottfried said, "After I began to realize my faults, I have been faithful with my tooth brush and powder, without any one urging me to do so. After these results, I have turned a new leaf in my life . . . and many people are doing the same thing. This will also change the whole history, and not many years from now, all the people of the world will be doing the same thing as the Marion Dental Class has been doing."[16]

The Idea of Dental Hygiene

Among her other merits, young Lillian Gottfried was a keen spotter of trends. The Marion School program, which burst onto the American scene roughly concomitant with the founding of several other prominent dental hygiene programs, would indeed prove a model for oral hygiene regimens in which generations of public school students in the United States would be enrolled. Within a decade or so, many more state and local dental societies, usually working in collaboration with public schools, established dental hygiene programs for children consisting of some combination of prophylaxis, remedial treatment, and health education. Private citizens and governments cooperated in the building of several much-heralded dental clinics or dispensaries. The dentists who worked in these programs were typically paid to do so, but the services they provided were often free to patients—and particularly to those who were poor.

Lillian Gottfried did not need special perceptiveness to make such an accurate guess. All around the country, and particularly in urban public schools like Lillian's, public health reformers of the early twentieth century implemented programs designed to reduce the burden of disease and death associated with personal and environmental uncleanliness.[17] Indeed, the children of the Marion School already participated in medical inspections intended to halt the spread of communicable diseases like measles, ringworm, and lice. Programs like the Marion School's medical screening system targeted children, especially the children of poor immigrants, partly because children were considered more likely than their parents to be successfully assimilated into American life. Freedom from dental pain and the disability it caused seemed to dentists to be essential to this end, as did conformity with American aesthetic and hygienic standards and resultant opportunities in professional and private life. Dentists often referred to the characteristics of "confidence and self-respect" as being particularly American, and emphasized that by enhancing one's looks and health, proper dental care could maximize these attributes and thereby make dental patients better Americans. Describing a dental dispensary program in Rochester, New York, for example, one dentist noted that "Quite a number of the applicants are the children of our foreign population. We are helping to make them better citizens, better men and women. The care of the teeth is a step toward the care of the body in general, and with it increased confidence and self-respect."[18]

Americans of the early twentieth century vigorously debated the responsibilities of government for the welfare of citizens, and frequently expressed the fear that too much government largesse would "pauperize" adults, making them unwilling or unable to provide for themselves. At the same time, however, Americans usually supported—or could be pressured into supporting—programs that provided for young people, who were not expected to be economically self-sufficient, and who were increasingly excluded from paid labor in this period. The "gospel of wealth" promoted by Andrew Carnegie and other notable philanthropists of the early twentieth century taught that charitable resources were most wisely directed toward those who might yet turn themselves into productive citizens. Universal public schooling itself proceeded from this notion, epitomizing the idea that it was important to equip impressionable youth with the skills and knowledge necessary to achieve economic independence and participate in democracy.[19]

School dental hygiene programs reflected this mixed set of ideas about responsibility, which also animated the 1912 establishment of the US government's Children's Bureau, and, later, the Sheppard-Towner Infancy and Maternity Protection Act, both of which focused on providing health screening and education to the worthy poor. Unlike physicians, who successfully lobbied to restrict such programs from providing medical treatment, dentists did not generally oppose the direct provision of free care to children. Rather, the creation of a new category of care—the regular dental cleaning—reflected their professional consensus that American children's dental health was an asset not just of individual children, but of the community itself. "In this land of the brave, where all are supposed to be born 'free and equal,'" one writer asked, "have not these children a *right* to free dental service?"[20]

Though parallel programs existed in some American factories, most public and private dental hygiene programs did make children their primary clients. Though the political impetus for selecting children rather than adults for free hygiene services was powerful, there were also important medical and logistical reasons for this choice of the school as a site for the delivery of care. The biology of tooth formation and eruption played a role: youngsters of six or seven years of age were the new owners of teeth that would have to serve them for the rest of their lives, and dentists believed strongly that early intervention would best help to ensure that outcome. School hygiene programs, like programs of school-based medical inspection, also maximized the potential of compulsory school attendance to put children in contact with dental care providers.

Dentists eager for an opportunity to impress the importance of dentistry on American youth viewed the public school as the ideal medium for the transmission of that message. Schoolchildren were massed together, away from the pernicious influences of their home lives, for six or more hours per day, and were already encouraged to regard the school as an authoritative institution equal to or exceeding the church or the family. School medical inspection invited children to regard their schools as places of valuable modern information about physical health—and this was information they were unlikely to acquire at home. "As we cannot reach the home circles effectively through contact . . . and cannot educate the parent to educate the child, why not properly instruct the child in the schools?" one dentist asked.[21] Dentists thought of the leveling influence of American public schools as both medium and message. "Whatever we wish to see introduced in the life of a nation, we must first remember, must first be introduced into its schools. The school is the one force to unify all conditions of society," a Maryland dentist reflected.

Though there was an inexorable logic to school hygiene programs' focus on children, the success of such enterprises was by no means assured. To begin with, even among dentists, the idea that brushing, flossing, and having one's teeth professionally cleaned could reduce the rate of dental decay and contribute to one's general health was not widely accepted in the early twentieth century. Many dentists considered what was in the teeth (their chemical makeup, whether figured as a function of genetics or of maternal and childhood diet) to be much more important than what was on them. Though most dentists accepted that both factors were significant enough to warrant attention, some leaned much more strongly in one direction than in the other. For instance, one dentist who considered both possibilities argued that he did not "imagine that dietary treatment will ever be as important a factor in this work as will the manual cleaning and the chemical treatment."[22]

Even some dentists who applauded public oral hygiene programs had doubts about the wildly optimistic claims made for them. One Philadelphia dentist opined that "Clean mouths and well-cared-for teeth will not make scholars and angels of dullards and wayward children; neither will it lessen the tax-payer's burdens."[23]

School physicians shared this skepticism about oral hygiene, and there-fore omitted it from their medical inspection programs. One of the factors that first roused dentists to the cause of publicly funded school dental hygiene programs was the fact that screening systems to reduce the prevalence of communicable diseases like measles, lice, and ringworm paid no heed to the state of children's teeth. Dentists were exasperated by physicians' reluc-tance to include tooth decay on the list of conditions for which screening was performed. A small minority of dentists believed that the bacteria pres-ent in decayed teeth were infectious, and could be spread from one child to another in the environment of the schoolroom. No dentist doubted that dental decay, whether communicable or not, posed a continuing threat to the overall health of the affected child, and that physicians who ignored it were danger-ously shortsighted. The Marion School itself had had a medical inspector for more than three years when the dental inspection program was inaugurated. He had, the school principal said, obtained "marvelous results," but, as the continued presence of ill health and discipline problems among the Marion Squad members suggested, and as dentists themselves pointed out, not quite marvelous enough.[24]

At the turn of the century, dentists also bemoaned their federal, state, and local governments' relative inattention to the problems of dental health. "While the need for government attention to dentistry as a public health mea-sure may seem clear to all those who, from a knowledge of the facts, realize its importance, there are still some who for reasons best known to themselves turn a deaf ear to the suggestions which in the interest of humanity are made by those who foresee the results of this apathy," an editorial in *The Dental Cosmos* mourned in 1902.[25] Governments that realized the importance of den-tal care, dentists speculated, could also reap significant savings in tax dollars by reducing truancy and the need for children to repeat grades in school, as well as by producing self-sufficient citizens who would require less help from the state or from private charities in adulthood.

Finally, most Americans simply did not believe that the cleanliness and health of their teeth were matters of urgent concern. Except among the well-to-do, daily brushing and flossing were uncommon practices. Dentists complained constantly that their patients were prone to demand extraction over fillings or root canals, and to refuse to pay the low cost of prophylaxis because they simply didn't consider their teeth worth the money. One writer estimated that "regarding only those who systematically and regularly have their teeth cared for by a dentist, we have from five to eight percent of our entire population. . . . [People] could, and would, find the means to pay for dental work, if they fully realized its importance. Its necessity had not been sufficiently impressed on their minds."[26]

Attempts by dentists to convince everyday Americans of the importance of good dental care reflected dentists' sense of the urgency of the task. These efforts also illustrated dentists' disregard for the privacy and autonomy of their educational targets and sometimes backfired as a result, adding to the opposition hygiene programs faced. The dentists who worked in the Marion School scorned the religious beliefs, base occupations, and living conditions of their young patients' parents. The members of the Marion School Dental Squad, nearly all of whom were Jewish, were identified in several widely distributed dental journals by their full names. Dentists who described these patients argued that the notorious parsimony and superstitiousness of Jews hindered the students' success. Frank Silverstein's father was "a tailor, not busy all the time"; the dental hygienist who visited Rose Lieberman's house had "considerable difficulty in persuading the mother not to give her sloppy food."[27] Dentist William Ebersole, in describing one Marion School student, noted that "the home is small and dirty; the family is large, the mother not strong, and seems unable to take proper care of her children. They are surrounded by an atmosphere of fear and superstition."[28] Another pupil he judged as "unreliable and careless. There was nothing in the home to help her, her mother being sickly, nervous and superstitious, throwing about the children the worst kind of atmosphere."[29] Several journals reprinted photographs of the Marion School children's homes and neighborhoods, highlighting the students' poverty and the seediness of their surroundings. School hygiene programs encouraged children to rise above such constraints and defy their superstitious, unscientific immigrant parents. The supervising hygienist of a program in Locust Point, Maryland, wrote amusedly that "one little chap told his teacher that when his mother, thinking him asleep, closed his window, he always got up quietly and raised it again; another that now that the kitchen seemed so hot and stuffy, she wrapped up and sat out in the back yard to get air."[30] Though the parents of Marion School students seemed to appreciate dentists' ministrations to their children, such outside innovations often sparked struggle and resentment between immigrant children and their parents—and prompted some parents to refuse to cooperate with reform programs.[31]

Nevertheless, dentists thought that school hygiene programs could help to persuade immigrant children and their parents of the importance of dental care. Their motives for seizing on American public schools as sites for dental education were technological, logistical, and political, but they were also entrepreneurial. Many advocates saw school hygiene programs as a way to lead American schoolchildren into an adult life of spending on privately provided, privately paid-for dental care. Though "ethical" dentists agreed that individual advertising was unprofessional, and frequently scorned those who engaged in it, most also agreed that advertising the concept of preventative dentistry would be acceptable. School dental programs provided an important forum for the professionally appropriate drumming-up of future business.

Dentists believed that the dissemination of information about proper dental hygiene might strengthen not only individual dentists' chances of winning patients, but the prestige of the profession itself: they linked their interest in school hygiene programs to their ongoing struggle to purge their ranks of slackers and establish their vocation as a high-status profession. They evinced a profound trust in the force of demand from an educated public to accomplish the regulation of their profession. Though school dental hygiene programs were the cornerstones of the hygiene education efforts, public-service style advertisements in newspapers and magazines also played a role.[32] "A public thus educated will demand intelligent, capable, scientific dentists, and will also elevate the standard of the profession," one writer mused.[33] Another hoped that if the public were better educated about dentistry, "the cry for cheap work would cease. The conditions which make the reign of the charlatan and quack would no longer exist. He would thus be either whipped into line or relegated to the rear. The splendid results would replenish our ranks with the choicest personnel from the scientific realm."[34] Some dentists professed to have heard colleagues comment that they "did not want the people to be possessed of knowledge in regard to teeth":[35] the implication was always that such reluctant individuals, perhaps from a previous generation of dentists who lacked thorough college training, feared for a professional status to which they were not entitled anyway. Few detractors raised their voices at the meetings of major dental organizations: the consensus reflected in both published articles and transcribed meeting proceedings was that the more patients knew about their own teeth, the more they would demand the services of ethical dentists, and that this was an outcome devoutly to be hoped for.

Dentists sought to parlay the rising entrance standards of the profession, as well as the high status of contemporary science and widespread popular knowledge of new scientific discoveries, into national consensus about the essential importance of good dental hygiene. New knowledge about germ theory and the importance of personal cleanliness to avoiding infection figured heavily in dentists' attempts to impress upon their patients, the public, and various levels of government the importance of having consistently (sometimes professionally) cleaned teeth. Many argued to their colleagues that dentists ought to present oral hygiene as a logical extension of other personal habits: "You would not sit down to breakfast without washing your hands and face," one dentist claimed to have told his patients, "and yet your mouth is dirtier than your hands or face. If you had not time to wash your mouth you had not time to wash your hands and face, as one is as necessary as the other."[36] Writers who advocated a focus on the bacterial origins of the bad smells coming from early twentieth-century children hoped to build on other public-health successes, like the construction of human waste and insects as dirty items that civilized people abhorred and disposed of as quickly as possible.[37] "The mores will eventually change until the unclean, uncared-for mouth will be considered as much of a popular menace as the open privy vault, the filthy garbage can, and the unswatted fly," one man wrote. He argued that existing public health powers ought to be applied to the problem of dental hygiene: "Individuals have no more right to maintain their mouths in a filthy condition than they have to throw bedroom slops into the street."[38] Even dentists who did not agree that bacteria, rather than oral filth itself, caused dental disease concurred that the habits of personal cleanliness that had already been successfully inculcated in many Americans—like hand washing, use of sanitary toilets, and refraining from spitting in public—would help to solve the problem of tooth decay, if Americans could be persuaded to extend those habits to their teeth. "What has been done in the treatment of zymotic diseases, namely, an improvement in the condition of surroundings, is precisely what is required respecting the teeth," US Navy dentist Richard Grady argued.[39]

Early twentieth-century schools were filthy places. "The building and the pupils must be clean," one physician wrote, "Send the children home if they smell, and clean the building by the vacuum system. In most schools a cloud of dust rises about three feet from the floor when the children run or dance on it." Other writers casually offered testimony as to why schools were in such bad condition: even in Bridgeport, Connecticut, a thriving manufacturing city in this period, "no public school has hot water, and few have gas or electric lights," reported one observer.[40] Turn-of-the-century classrooms were, as a result, veritable hotbeds of miasma: "Have you ever frequented the schoolroom and not had your olfactories set your thought factory in motion as to the origin of the peculiar aroma in the atmosphere?" one dentist demanded. "That aroma is largely caused by the exhalation of air through the oral and nasal cavities and over their foul surfaces; it is freighted with the very poison that, when it finds lodgement in fertile soil, precipitates the occasional epidemics of children's diseases."[41] Another wrote: "Several teachers in the primary grades have told me that even on the coldest days in winter it is impossible to close the windows for five minutes on account of the odor from the children's bodies."[42] Some writers suggested that children's bad breath ought to be treated as evidence of a communicable disease, causing children to be excluded from school until the odor had disappeared. "Parents will send the children to school with their faces clean, if it is demanded," one dentist wrote, "Why should they not send them with clean mouths so that the neighbor's child will not have to breathe the vile atmosphere resulting from rows of decaying teeth and abscessed roots?"[43] Repeated reports of noxious smells in public-school classrooms provided an opportunity to link the old understanding of the toxicity of bad smells with the new knowledge that it was germs that caused those odors, and suggested that the schoolroom would be an important site at which dentists could establish in the popular mind the importance of good dental hygiene.

Dentists also hoped to rely upon patients' vanity to sell dental services, including professional cleanings and instruction in home care. Complaining that many patients demanded that carious teeth be extracted rather than filled, and seemed not to regard the loss of a tooth as problematic, California dentist Russell Cool argued that "We should remind them that the loss of a tooth has its effect upon the expression of the face; that it influences the alignment of the other teeth; and that it destroys part of the vocal apparatus."[44] Over time, more dentists noted that in encouraging patients to seek regular dental care, "the most salient force, both in working among children and adults, was impressing the close relationship the subject had to question of personal beauty."[45] Dentists who made aesthetic arguments for dental hygiene were not simply emphasizing the factor they felt was most likely

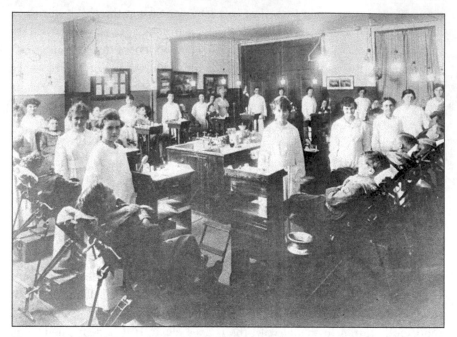

Figure 1 Alfred Fones's second class of dental hygienists, performing cleanings on Boy Scouts. *Dental Digest* 34 (May 1928): 323.

to sway image-conscious patients: Russell Cool, for one, could rhapsodize at length about "How often [we have], when charmed by a classic face that, in repose, excited admiration on account of the symmetry and regularity of the features and the purity of the skin, had this charm dispelled and a feeling of loathing induced as a smile revealed, instead of the expected pearls, a shocking array of blackened and crumbling snags, or tawdry and self-assertive gold fillings."[46] In fact, some dentists believed that keeping one's teeth clean and in good repair could actually improve one's looks overall: if advice about the care of the teeth were widely disseminated, one dentist speculated, "there would be less need of so-called beauty hints as to the care of pimples and facial blemishes."[47] He, like the advocates of the Cleveland and Marion School hygiene campaigns, specifically linked the good looks that could be ensured through good dental hygiene with success in life: "We can, if permitted, teach them that soundness of teeth is one of the best evidences of general soundness of body; that the care of the teeth pays in comfort, in beauty, in the conservation of health; that the care of the teeth tells of inborn politeness, and sustains association with well-bred men and women."[48]

Dentists formed a thriving coalition around the concept of oral hygiene. Debates about the influence of other factors, particularly diet and genetics, on tooth decay would continue to rage more or less simultaneously with the struggle to initiate publicly funded oral hygiene programs for children. But by the time of the Marion School program almost no dentists—and, at least as dentists told it, few properly educated laypeople—seriously doubted that keeping one's teeth clean could have a positive impact on one's health and appearance. Nor did they doubt that encouraging that cleanliness, and the personal qualities that came with it, could be an important part of campaigns to Americanize immigrants, particularly immigrant children. Dentists' growing professional authority and the success of their attempts to market the idea of preventative dental care resulted in millions of tax dollars being spent to establish dental hygiene programs in public schools—and millions of private dollars to found free or low-cost dental clinics. As early as 1902, *The Dental Cosmos* jubilantly published a long list of "efforts in behalf of disseminating oral-hygienic knowledge in schools," which were being made by an impressive array of state and local dental societies, as well as by the National Dental Association itself—often, as in the Marion School, with the cooperation of school authorities.[49] Several school dental programs, including those of the Rochester, New York, public schools and one paid for by the Children's Aid Society of New York City, received extensive coverage in dental journals.[50]

Private Dental Philanthropy

In their native Boston and around the country, the generosity of the Forsyth family received almost as much publicity as did any public clinic, perhaps because the family's magnanimity enabled the establishment of a dental facility far in excess of even the loftiest aspirations of most public programs. The benefactors of the clinic were a group of brothers, one of whom, James Bennet Forsyth, had attempted to make provisions for the clinic in his will before he died in 1900; the document was later (for reasons that were not elaborated upon in dental journals) declared void. Two of his surviving brothers, John Hamilton and James Alexander Forsyth, decided to pursue their deceased brother's dream of founding a clinic to care for the children of the worthy poor. The deceased brother, as they told it, had "had considerable trouble with his teeth. The doctors who attended him told him if they had received proper care during his childhood days they would have saved him considerable pain and trouble."[51] James Bennet Forsyth had planned to give $500,000 of his considerable personal fortune to the clinic: John Hamilton and James Alexander Forsyth tripled the sum.[52]

The Forsyth Infirmary, which opened in 1915, was a veritable palace of dentistry. The Forsyth brothers—and the editor of *The Dental Brief*—pointed out that since the building was intended to serve both as a dental clinic and as a memorial to James Bennet Forsyth, "the building on this account embodies many artistic features usually lacking in buildings intended solely for hospital purposes."[53] The children's waiting room, for example, contained an aquarium of native fish, multiple artistic panels illustrating some classic children's tales (including "Rip Van Winkle" and "The Pied Piper"), and a "well selected juvenile library," in addition to tile floors, ceilings, and walls, which could be "flushed with a hose from top to bottom, thus ensuring sanitation and cleanliness."[54] The main operatory had sixty-four fully equipped dental chairs and room for forty more; there was a separate "extraction room," as well as a clinic "devoted to nose, throat and ear operations."[55] The "marble-faced clocks" in each room were "controlled by the master clock in the director's room."[56] The building also featured a research laboratory and an amphitheater that seated two hundred and fifty people: it was intended for public lectures on oral hygiene, but it could also be used for the instruction of dental students and clinicians and, owing to its tile construction, could be flushed with "live steam or water after each operation."[57]

Public and professional response to the majestic infirmary building was no less grandiose than the edifice itself. The editor of *Oral Hygiene* recommended that the fortunate trustees of the elaborate new building "should enter on their duties with prayer and fasting," as befit men who were taking on such important roles in the public service.[58] At the dedication of the clinic on November 24, 1914, the mayor of Boston pointed out that the new Forsyth clinic demonstrated the contrast between American values (of "toil, thrift, and love of humanity") and those of "the other side of the Atlantic" (where World War I had just begun, and where "men are engaged in the destruction of human life"). He declared that the clinic "should so tend to change the current of public thought as to cause its donors, the Forsyth brothers, to outrank in the estimation of thinking men and women the greatest warriors of our time."[59] Charles Eliot, president emeritus of nearby Harvard University, argued that the clinic "illustrates one of the admirable traits of the successful business men in the United States—the desire on their part to make use of their private earnings and accumulations to advance some beneficial public undertaking."[60] Thomas Forsyth, another Forsyth brother who would serve

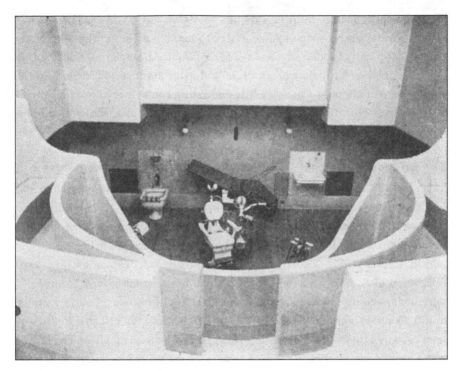

Figure 2   The amphitheater in the Forsyth dental clinic, 1914. *Oral Hygiene* 5 (January 1915): 15.

as a trustee of the clinic, explicitly articulated his hopes for a public benefit from the clinic: he wanted children to be healthier and happier, and "by making them healthier and happier I hope it may make them grow to be better citizens of our beloved Boston."[61]

The Forsyth clinic was, therefore, a marker not only of the objective importance of dental hygiene to good health, but of a confluence of individual and national qualities and aspirations that were slowly but steadily becoming attached to the concept of dental hygiene. The clinic enabled a wealthy family to demonstrate its philanthropic bent by funding a forward-thinking enterprise, the presence of which "should change the current of public thought" toward a greater appreciation of both oral hygiene and the Forsyth brothers themselves. It became a place for the construction of an imputed set of shared national values—"toil, thrift, and love of humanity"—and a vision of citizenship that took health and happiness as necessary prerequisites for becoming "better citizens of our beloved Boston." Most importantly to dentists, however, by addressing Boston children's dental needs on such a magnificent scale, the clinic elevated the status of dentistry to make it a peer of the other great philanthropically funded needs of the early twentieth century—Andrew Carnegie's libraries, for instance, which in a similar manner acknowledged the importance of citizens' literacy while endorsing the values of toil and thrift. As the editor of *Oral Hygiene* gushed: "It is an uplift to the whole dental profession throughout the world."[62]

The Bridgeport Campaign and the Birth of the Dental Hygienist

Though the Forsyth clinic and the Marion School hygiene campaign did much to draw lay and professional attention to the cause of dental hygiene, no events in dentistry would attract as much interest as the establishment of a comprehensive, publicly funded dental hygiene program in Bridgeport, Connecticut, in 1914. The scale of the enormous Bridgeport campaign forced the resolution of an issue that dentists had been debating for at least ten years—whether specially trained women, rather than highly educated male dentists, could be relied upon to do the rote work of cleaning Americans' teeth. The lead organizer of the Bridgeport campaign, a dentist named Alfred Fones, had already incurred the scorn of his colleagues for having suggested, in several professional meetings and published articles, that women could be trained to do dental hygiene work without undergoing a complete dental education. Detractors feared that allowing anyone but a properly trained dentist to take on responsibility for Americans' teeth would damage the professional status for which dentists were still fighting. What constituted "proper" training was anything but well-established in the 1910s, adding to the anxiety for those who opposed the idea of the woman hygienist. Fones's enormous personal magnetism and the success of the ten-year Bridgeport hygiene program nevertheless produced a new professional role for women who might otherwise have been nurses, social workers, or teachers, and a new challenge for dentists to contend with: the existence of the dental hygienist.

Alfred Fones was a native of Bridgeport. His father, Civilion Fones, had been a remarkably well-trained dentist for his time (he graduated from the Baltimore College of Dentistry in 1873), and Alfred followed in his footsteps, graduating from the New York University College of Dentistry in 1890.[63] In 1899, at a meeting of the Northeastern Dental Association, Fones heard a Philadelphia dentist give a talk on what he referred to as "controlled practice": he required his patients to visit him at regular intervals for professional care and to clean their own teeth regularly at home.[64] Fones was immediately persuaded by the genius of the Philadelphian's system, which allowed for preventive care instead of emergency repairs and resulted in more patients retaining more of their teeth until late in life. However, Fones was troubled by the one factor that seemed to militate against its widespread implementation: professional dentists had increasingly become too well educated to spend their valuable hours in the mindless (and low-paying) repetition of cleaning teeth, and patients would not pay for cleaning at rates that would make the task worth dentists' time. Furthermore, if every American was to be placed on a schedule of regular dental hygiene, there could never be enough dentists to meet the projected need, particularly as barriers to entry into the profession grew ever higher.

Like many dentists of his time, Fones had long employed a woman assistant (also known as a "chair nurse" or "dental nurse") to do his scheduling and billing, greet patients, and assist him at the dental chair. He reasoned that the repetitive work of dental hygiene fell well within the limits of responsibility that dental assistants had already assumed, and decided to train his own assistant to perform hygiene treatments, which she did for the first time in 1906.[65] Over a period of several years, he discharged from his practice patients who were unwilling to follow a regular schedule of dental hygiene treatments, until everyone who was left was having his or her teeth cleaned every two months. Fones calculated that having his assistant regularly clean his patients' teeth actually saved both his own time and patients' money: specifically, he figured that his hygiene plan cost patients 40 percent as much as seeking dental treatment on an as-needed basis.[66] On the other hand, because he could maintain a larger roster of patients who needed less intensive care, Fones's own patient volume—and his income—rose during the same period.

Fones's plan for training and using dental hygienists, which he articulated in many professional forums before successfully implementing it in the Bridgeport schools, was a controversial one. The dental assistant had long been constructed, both by dentists and by assistants themselves, as a sort of office wife: she served the dentist's interests, not her own, and she worked entirely under his direction and at his pleasure. Her role was to provide a buffer between the dentist and the more painful realities of entrepreneurial individualism—the need to pursue patients who failed to pay, do business with dental-supply salespeople, and deal with patients who insisted on too much of the dentist's time, or who developed inappropriate hypochondriacal attachments to their dentists. Alternatively, she could play the role of the office mother—greeting and serving as a hostess to patients, ensuring the comfort of children whom the dentist might not be totally comfortable treating, and (as Juliette Southard, the founder of the professional dental assistant's organization pointed out) by her own sterling presence, serving as a guarantee against charges of sexual misconduct by the dentist.[67] Though such charges were uncommon, the possibility was of particular concern to dentists who practiced alone in private office settings.

The hygienist, on the other hand, was something of an unknown quantity. Dentists who wanted to be able to hire hygienists to work in their own offices, or who favored having hygienists instead of dentists do the day-to-day work of school and industrial hygiene programs, argued that women were better suited than men to the fine, repetitive, mundane handwork required for hygiene treatments. (If this contradicted the frequent claim that women lacked the mechanical aptitude needed to make them successful dentists, the practitioners who advocated for the role of the dental hygienist did not notice it.) Some dentists had hired newly trained male "graduate dentists" as junior partners and the primary providers of hygiene in their offices, only to find that these overly ambitious male colleagues broke ranks and started their own offices after a few years—sometimes within a competitive distance of their prior employer's own shop. Women, advocates of the trained dental hygienist argued, would be less prone to want independence. They could actually be legally restrained from seeking it by narrowly crafted—usually sex-specific—hygiene practice acts that prevented hygienists from working without the supervision of a dentist. The trained "dental nurse," like a medical nurse, would clean body parts in preparation for the ministrations of the doctor or dentist; there seemed, to advocates of the hygienist model, to be ample precedent for her presence in the dental office.

From the hygienist's first appearance on the scene, however, dentists feared the effect that the existence of trained women hygienists would have on their own professional fortunes. Some doubted that truly intelligent, well-trained hygienists would be happy being restrained from performing more complicated operations that were technically within the province of the dentist himself: "How could we ever give a legal standing to such persons, to keep whom within the limits of their proper functions would probably be a continual source of trouble?" asked University of Michigan dentist Neville Hoff in 1912.[68] Hoff, among others, feared that the elision of the boundary between dentist and trained dental nurse would serve the cause of quackery, dragging the status of the profession down with it: "Would not the advertising quacks use this open door to fill their offices with unskilled and unlettered employees, with greater injury to the people and to the utter confusion of our professional standards?" he demanded.[69] Ironically, the most vigorous opponents of the hygienist concept were those who placed the most stock in women's ambitions—for the greater such ambitions were, the higher the likelihood that women hygienists would overstep their boundaries and do harm to dentists' professional status.

Like female physicians who preferred to work without nursing assistance, the few women dentists who had struggled successfully to get professional standing were among the loudest critics of the notion of bringing lesser-trained auxiliaries into an office setting. Hygienist advocates sometimes claimed that the work of cleaning teeth, like the work of cleaning hair or fingernails, was not sufficiently difficult to require much professional training, but, as Detroit dentist Grace Rogers complained, they offered no explanation for why a self-respecting woman would spend a year or more being trained to hold "an irresponsible position."[70] "What object would any young woman have in spending so much time in fitting herself for such an occupation?" Rogers asked "She would have but one, and that, a higher salary than a person with her qualifications could demand in any other position."[71]

Tensions around money and professionals' proper relationship to it underlay much of the debate about the role of the dental hygienist. Though dentists recognized the collection of fees as an important part of their practices, they categorized financial management as falling outside their own professional purview, which was precisely why so many of them preferred to have dental assistants attend to their accounts. Suspicions ran high of those who admitted to having entered the profession—or any profession—for money, and Grace Rogers's concern about the pecuniary motives of hygienists resonated quite strongly with practitioners of the time. One opponent of the dental hygienist specifically noted that all of the hygienists who had trained at the Forsyth Infirmary had entered private practice rather than "the field of charity," and that the private dentists who employed them made great—and therefore suspicious—profits from their work. Another dentist wrote to *The Dental Cosmos* the following month to dispute this claim, but did not challenge the premise that aspirations to financial success would have been inappropriate, particularly for professional women. The director of a dispensary in Rochester that trained hygienists claimed that 45 percent of them went on to work in public institutions. "I have preferred to send graduates to public rather than to private institutions," he wrote, "because I have felt that their work would demonstrate to the public the value of oral prophylaxis and in that way stimulate public authorities to make larger appropriations for dental work."[72] Income differentials within the profession of dentistry itself also sparked resentment, and opposition to the dental hygienist: one New Jersey dentist pointed out that the dentists who were the strongest advocates for the use of trained dental nurses were also those with the largest and most lucrative practices. "Granting, for the sake of argument, that the dental nurse, fulfilling her duties in a proper manner, would be ideal; how many of the men practicing dentistry in the United States could afford to employ such a nurse? Most of them would be well content to be kept busy themselves . . ." he observed.[73]

Hygiene and Americanism

Dentists who sought to build consensus within the profession about the merits of oral hygiene drew upon a vast popular and professional knowledge of the importance of Americanizing, by flattery or by force, the hundreds of thousands of immigrants who flocked to the United States each year before the passage of national laws restricting immigration. This generally meant persuading immigrants of the necessity of adopting white Protestant norms of health, hygiene, cookery, gender behavior, business interaction and school attendance, among other facets of early twentieth-century life in the United States. An increasingly large and sophisticated infrastructure, both public and private, emerged to accomplish this task. This apparatus, like the dental hygiene programs dentists advocated, was usually staffed by middle- to upper-class women, who were believed to be particularly effective transmitters of cultural values, and who frequently welcomed the opportunity to find paid employment outside the home.

The debate about whether women should be trained as dental hygienists, whether and how the law should recognize them as licensed professionals in their own right, and in what settings their services should be employed reflected dentists' fears and hopes for their profession. However, it also demonstrated dentists' sense that dentistry had something important to add to a national discussion about what health practices could be regarded as "American." One faction, skeptical that hygienists could be kept from encroaching on dentists' own turf and fearing for the impact of "unlettered" women doing dental work on the status of the profession, opposed the training and licensing of hygienists. Advocates of this position also feared that in popularizing dental hygiene as a means of Americanization, dentists might inadvertently contribute to a dangerous corruption of American dental care. This group thus opposed publicly funded dental hygiene programs, which they constructed as un-American. "Does anyone believe that you could train and equip at the present-day low standard of educational requirements a sufficient number of dental hygienists to give personal care to the teeth of all children . . . and all of this to be at public expense? That is a thought 'made in Germany,' and much resembles paternalism and German 'kultur' and not at all likely in this or any other state," argued one Massachusetts dentist in 1919.[74]

Another faction hoped that public dental hygiene programs would increase the demand for high-quality dental care and thereby increase the status of the profession. They believed that such programs could not be carried out without the aid of trained hygienists, and maintained an ebullient optimism about the potential of publicly funded dental hygiene programs to serve as agents of Americanization for immigrants without endangering American dental care itself. They rejected the accusation that such beliefs and aspirations were un-American and actively promoted the dental hygienist as an instrument by which foreigners could be inculcated with Americanism. "In the mining districts of Luzerne County [Pennsylvania] hundreds of foreigners are employed. I would like some of the opponents of the oral hygienist to examine the mouths of these foreigners before the oral hygienist had treated them, and then examine them again after her work was finished. It would be a revelation to them," one Pennsylvania dentist opined. "The children are so anxious to learn and take advantage of any opportunity given them, and I know that a clean mouth and a talk on hygiene has started many of them on the right road to good American citizenship."[75]

Both factions agreed that increasing the status of the profession and promoting good citizenship were important goals, and saw those goals as being inextricably linked. But they differed in their ideas about how to achieve those goals, and about how to define a properly American dental care policy. Ultimately, opponents of the dental hygienists and the programs they staffed were outnumbered, outgunned, and resoundingly trounced. The process of legalizing the professional practice of dental hygienists was carried out state by state, took several decades, and provided frequent opportunities for dentists at state and national conferences to object to the idea of the trained dental nurse. Not coincidentally, however, the prolonged nature of the campaign to legalize the role of the dental hygienist also provided multiple opportunities for those who objected to the concept to have their resistance softened by the smashing success of the hygienist-run programs. One measure of the prevailing point of view can be had in the 1922 decision of the American Dental

Association to encourage dental hygienists, dental assistants, and dental laboratory technicians to form their own independent organizations.[76] Alfred Fones's Bridgeport hygiene campaign, among others, succeeded in swaying the predominant opinion within the profession in favor of the hygienist and all her works.

Fones, like other advocates of the dental hygienist concept, saw the Bridgeport hygiene program as merging dentistry's professional and civic goals almost flawlessly. As one chronicler of the Bridgeport campaign pointed out, Fones's father Civilion had been a member (and, for one year, the president) of the Connecticut State Dental Commission, the president of his state dental association, and a councilman, an alderman, and mayor of the city of Bridgeport.[77] The writer credited Civilion's background in public service for having spurred Alfred Fones's interest in applying the principles of his oral hygiene program to the schoolchildren of Bridgeport, a navy town whose large population of munitions workers was dense with recent immigrants. After several years of pestering local officials, Fones was able to convince the Bridgeport Board of Health to allocate funds for the initiation of a school hygiene program in 1914.[78] He was so confident of his eventual success that he had spent much of 1913 training the first group of women dental hygienists, who received lecture instruction from some of the most distinguished figures in contemporary dentistry. The hygienists spent their first year in practice moving from school to school, cleaning children's teeth, giving lectures on oral hygiene, and distributing educational materials for the parents of Bridgeport schoolchildren. In the second year of the campaign, a woman dentist also visited the schools, filling small cavities in children's first permanent molars. The next year, a second dentist was added.[79]

School officials placed a high priority on the Bridgeport campaign. Though, as one writer reported, "no public school [in Bridgeport] has hot water, and few have gas or electric lights," principals made extraordinary efforts to provide Fones and his hygienists with suitable locations in which to practice.[80] In fact, two principals gave up their offices to the hygiene program, moving their desks into corridors that were not light enough for hygiene work, and may well have been barely light enough for administration work.[81] Teachers, one hygienist said, "are eager to assist us in every way, questioning the children between our visit [sic] as to the use of their tooth-brushes; also the motions of the prescribed method of brushing."[82] At one school, the teachers' lounge was used for dental cleanings because it had a two-burner hot plate that could be used for boiling water to sterilize instruments.[83]

Bridgeport proved an excellent laboratory for one of the central theories of the oral hygiene movement—that children who were educated about the importance of dental hygiene could become, as one writer put it, "missionaries to the home," and to their larger communities, helping to inculcate the "Gospel of clean mouths" in a population sorely in need of this Americanizing message.[84] Like the Marion School program, the campaign produced many success stories in this regard, which were widely reported and repeated, more or less word for word, in several prominent dental journals. Children who had feared the dentist and hygienists, it was said, came to beg for dental work and place social premiums upon it. One boy, for instance, was reluctant to come to school when he had lost his toothbrush—perhaps because his teacher was the one who reportedly allowed her students the otherwise unheard-of luxury of clapping their hands "when everyone reports 'brushed teeth.'"[85] A "Jewish boy with a terrible mouth," after asking many questions about the oral hygiene program, recruited an entire clinic's worth of children to participate in the program on a Saturday morning.[86] In a vignette that suggested the somewhat brutal mores of the contemporary American schoolroom, one child who had failed to brush his teeth, when given a choice between going back to his classroom without his teeth professionally cleaned and receiving both a whipping and a hygiene treatment, chose the hygiene treatment. In the end, the benevolent hygienist dispensed with the whipping.[87] A group of older boys who thought that they might not receive hygiene treatments because of their advanced age broke into a storeroom in a Bridgeport school and stole two dozen toothbrushes, which the hygienists took not as evidence of the irremediable criminality of immigrants, but of their great—and justified—enthusiasm for dentistry.[88]

Similarly, parents who had been "too little educated to understand American ideals or to care about physical cleanliness"[89] appeared to hold dental care in renewed regard. Some immigrant children began to appear in the Bridgeport school clinics with privately obtained dental work, and the parents "told the teachers how the children are always brushing their teeth," though the hygienist who reported this gave no hint of whether the parents provided this information with pride or bafflement.[90] Others in the community, too, saw the good results of the children's hygiene treatments: a Bridgeport hygienist related that "during one of our visits to a large school in a thickly populated foreign district, one noon hour a small boy who had had his teeth cleaned that morning was seen sitting on the sidewalk surrounded by six or eight men, all talking and laughing in their excitable Italian way. On investigation it was found that the boy was holding his mouth open and turning his lips back to show how clean his teeth were, and the men were delighted with the results."[91] The posture in which the boy was holding his mouth was also the position children were required to hold in order to have their teeth cleaned. That the small boy might have been mocking the hygiene program rather than flaunting its results apparently did not occur to the hygienist who reported the story—or to the other writers who repeated it as evidence of the program's success in inculcating good hygienic values in immigrants.

Hygienists and dentists who reported on the successes of the Bridgeport hygiene program frequently cast ambiguous evidence in the best possible light, suggesting how thoroughly convinced they were that the wisdom of the oral hygiene campaign was obvious, both to them and to its subjects. Over time, propelled by this certainty and by the genuine acclaim the program received from school officials, the scope of the campaign grew: more hygienists were hired, and Fones successfully shepherded through the Connecticut state legislature enabling legislation giving dental hygienists legal recognition.[92] In 1917, Fones offered the services of the program to clean and repair the teeth of National Guardsmen who were stationed in Bridgeport awaiting their departure to join the Allied Expeditionary Forces in Europe, and the commanding officer took him up on the offer: Fones and his hygienists donated their services free of charge.[93] In the winter of 1918–1919, when many American schools closed because of the deadly influenza pandemic that swept across the United States that season, the schools in Bridgeport, "almost alone among big cities in the East," stayed open, and the city "recorded the lowest death rate of any city its size, 5.2 per 1000 people. The City Health Officer gave the teaching of the dental clinic great credit for this result."[94]

Dental Health as a National Asset

The centerpiece of dentists' attempts to inspire public interest in dental hygiene was their claim that because bad dental health could cause so many diseases and so much lost time from school and work—as the example of the 1918–1919 influenza epidemic demonstrated—the oral hygiene of citizens was properly of great concern not only to individual patients, but also to the state itself. "If bad teeth could be prevented," one dentist pointed out, "the gain to the State and the individual would be of enormous value, as it is wonderful how many diseases can be traced indirectly to bad teeth."[95] To contemporary observers, the stakes of the oral hygiene problem were extraordinarily high: some argued that when bad dental health resulted in time lost from school, the foundations of democracy were imperiled. "The whole theory of democracy," one man sputtered, "is built on the assumption that the voters shall be intelligent." He noted that some 250,000 children a year failed to achieve the contemporary standard of intelligence for democracy— graduation from the eighth grade—often because their progress in school had been retarded by poor health: "It is wasteful to the state and inhuman to the child to have his progress in school blocked because he has some removable defect," he opined.[96] Children who had to repeat grades in school cost tax-payers money: "The neglect of children's teeth is increasing the taxes of the United States many millions of dollars each year," asserted prominent Los Angeles pedodontist M. Evangeline Jordan.[97] Those who flunked out of school entirely remained burdens on the rest of society forever: "Neglected children are apt later in life to become unproductive citizens who must be taken care of by the productive units of society," one writer warned.[98] Some writers put the matter more directly: if the poor health of citizens were a drain on the state, then the propagation and maintenance of their good health must be a positive asset. "Every normal child is an asset to its parents and the Govern-ment, State and Federal, and every possible means of protecting and devel-oping this asset is worthy of our most careful consideration," said the Ohio governor's representative at the 1910 oral hygiene kickoff rally.[99]

Propaganda directed at children on this point proliferated in the early twentieth century. Dental hygiene training films were shown to young people in school and before feature films in movie theaters, and dentists circulated short stories and lectures to be delivered to school groups.[100] One genre in particular suggests the insistence with which dentists sought to propagate the notion that children and their dental care were matters of public concern: skits published in dental journals and intended for performance by children sought to enlist children as both audience for, and purveyor of, the message that healthy teeth and a healthy nation somehow went hand in hand. In 1913, for example, the journal *Oral Hygiene* published a skit in which the lead characters, to be played by preteen youngsters, were "Uncle Sam" and "Miss Columbia." The latter advised the audience that "if a deformed or unhealthy tooth or the loss of a tooth keeps a boy or girl out of school or makes their mouths a place for disease germs to grow fat in . . . Uncle Samuel cares."[101] Uncle Sam concurred: "We cannot afford to dally," he opined, "we must do something in every school district in the country."[102] The playlet anticipated the objections that dental care was secondary to medical care, that no health care ought to be provided through the public schools at all, or that physicians already working in the schools were adequately trained to diagnose and refer dental disease, and it introduced characters who addressed all of these concerns. "Dr. Medico" argued that "We medical doctors and our brothers in the profession, the dentists must work together for the public good and prevention is the key to success."[103] Teacher Miss Bright cited the favorable results of the Marion School dental study, while Rev. B. Earnest declaimed that "we cannot as Christian people fairly represent the Master who went about doing good to the bodies of men as well as to their souls, unless we come in closer sympathy with such work. I hope the day will come when every public school shall have dental supervision."[104] Miss Esthetic commented that "we see miracles every day in the straightening of teeth . . . resulting in better health and better looks."[105]

More than just trying to convince the skit's viewers of the need for government involvement in American children's dental care, the statement that "Uncle Sam cares" also embodied an existing truth. The success of the hygiene programs helped to make a reputation for concern about dental health, or at least for the existence of a thriving infrastructure dedicated to the promotion of it, an important piece of American national identity. The playlet magnified this connection in ways that would have seemed ludicrous had the link not been so widely recognized already. Directions to the stage manager included the suggestion that "A large American flag as a background [is] appropriate," and emphasized the proper placement of the singing of "America" in the piece ("If announcements or collection follow the playlet, omit 'America' until dismissal"[106]) and the appropriate accompaniment for the singing of the requisite patriotic song: "If the Star Spangled Banner or other patriotic song than America is chosen for closing, small flags attached to toothbrushes may be waved by the entire cast."[107] "Master T. Ache," a student, made an appearance to highlight the difficulty encountered by students in poor dental health in learning the civics lessons essential to American citizenship. "For pity's sake," he wails, "won't some one take this awful ache out o'my head?/ How do I know where the currents flow, or Hood from Poe or which is dead?/ What do I care what's in the air 'r what rocks are bare in Idaho?/ What can I do in school or pew?/ It's up to you, unless you cage me in the zoo!"[108]

Programs of dental education and prophylaxis both reflected and contributed to the idea that the fate of the nation was somehow inextricably connected to the teeth of its people. Dentists pointed proudly to evidence that the American public had come to accept the notion that children's teeth were, in some ways, the responsibility of the state: one *Brooklyn Eagle* editorial, reprinted in *The Dental Brief* in 1911, conceded that "All [school hygiene] work is totally at variance with the fundamental American idea that it is the business of parents to provide for their own children. . . . But the fact is that, whether we like it or not, we are accepting more and more the communistic notion that it is the business of all the people of the city to care for all the children of the city."[109] Another writer continued in the same theme in 1920: "If that is socialism," he thundered, "let us be quick to incorporate it in every political creed. I am more willing to believe it is Americanism, and that it was in the minds of the writers of our constitution when they prepared its preamble."[110] Early in the twentieth century, the efforts of dentists to improve the status of their profession helped to draw good dentistry and good citizenship closer together in the minds of Americans. But dentists' enthusiastic professional nationalism contrasted sharply with darker fears about the cause of Americans' bad dental health. The question of why Americans needed dental care so badly lurked just under the surface.

Chapter 2

Diet and the Dental Critique of American Life

"We Boast of Our Civilization, But We Starve Our Children"

The optimistic spirit that pervaded dentists' activism for dental hygiene programs masked a deeper, more pessimistic set of fears about what might be causing the alarming rate of tooth decay in the United States. Dentists believed that as much as 90 percent of Americans suffered from tooth decay, and that as much as half of that decay had never been diagnosed or treated by a dentist. Theories proliferated to explain why Americans were so prone to tooth decay, and to the sorts of total-body derangements of health that "focal infection" spreading from a tooth to the rest of the body could cause. Early in the century, the dentists who designed and staffed public hygiene programs typically attributed decay at least in part to the deleterious presence of food debris, and bacteria that grew within it, on teeth. Yet some of their peers had already come to the conclusion that while cleaning the teeth was important for a variety of reasons, it was not a reliable preventative of cavities. Something else—perhaps the nature of the debris itself, or the nature of the teeth upon which it accumulated—seemed to be exerting an independently controlling influence over the occurrence of tooth decay.

Some practitioners hypothesized that individuals' inherent genetic tendencies controlled their dental health. Others argued the cases for a variety of other causative mechanisms for tooth decay—excessive alkalinity of the diet and/or the saliva, inadequate consumption of calcium, phosphorus, or vitamin D, and, finally, the existence in the mouth of lactobacillus bacteria, which flourished in sugar and attacked "susceptible" teeth to create cavities. In short, dentists contemplating the problem of tooth decay in the first half of the twentieth century focused on two factors: what was in the teeth, and what was on them. Arbiters of these two viewpoints shared their sense that the prevalence of dental decay meant something bad about America. They differed in their assessment of whether or not that bad thing was remediable— and, if so, how.

Tooth Decay as Genetic Degeneration

The preeminent theorist of genetic causes of tooth decay was Eugene Solomon Talbot, a Chicago dentist who had entered dental practice as an apprentice in 1870 and subsequently undertook a full course of medical training, graduating from Rush Medical College in 1880. In the debate among dentists about how to raise the status of the profession, Talbot was a lifetime advocate of "stomatology," which posited that dentists ought to imagine themselves as practitioners of a medical subspecialty focused on the mouth. Talbot's interest in human heredity, and his belief in its power, were widely shared in the early twentieth century not only by other physicians and dentists but by sociologists (and particularly criminologists), psychologists, and politicians.[1] Talbot, however, believed that dentists had something special to contribute to the science of inheritance, because he believed that human teeth were among the most sensitive markers of constitutional deterioration: in 1896, he wrote that "the ear should be the most frequently affected by degeneracy; next . . . come the jaws and teeth, and finally the head and face. Abnormal development of all is strong evidence of degeneracy."[2]

Like other practitioners of his time, Talbot stood in a constantly changing stream of knowledge about human heredity, and held accordingly complicated opinions about what traits could properly be classified as hereditary, the mechanisms by which hereditary traits were transmitted, and what counted as "degeneration" in the human body. "A degenerate, scientifically," Talbot said, "is a person whose brain and nervous system is unstable from inherited or acquired taint in the parents, who has in consequence undergone imperfectly the embryologic changes to a higher type in tissues or organs, and therefore exhibits tendencies liable to extinguish the race, as a type, under the usual conditions of the struggle for existence."[3] Unlike his contemporary, noted phrenologist and criminologist Cesar Lombroso, Talbot did not believe that degenerates constituted a separate race. Rather, he theorized that any individual deprived of two healthy parents, a minimum threshold of nutrition before birth, and careful medical care at all of the crises of life (including teething, puberty, and menopause) might develop weaknesses of the nervous system that would, in turn, affect all other structures and functions of the body, including the teeth.

Though degenerates, in Talbot's mind, were often beyond medical or moral redemption, degeneracy itself was not always a bad thing. Indeed, as the flawless dental health of many primitive peoples suggested to contemporary observers, perfect teeth could actually be a sign of inadequate evolutionary progress. Talbot believed that individual organs could degenerate for the benefit of their parent organism: as examples, he cited "the muscles of the ear, the vermiform appendix, the little toe, the false ribs, the pineal eye, but especially the face, including the nose, jaws, and teeth,"[4] which latter structures he believed to have deteriorated for the benefit of the human brain. Talbot speculated that the human fourth molars had evolved to extinction because nervous energy was required to more fully develop the human brain, thereby diverting that energy from the development of the teeth. He also believed that the fuller development of the nervous system meant that fewer teeth were required to do the chewing and digesting that man had craftily replaced with cooking and the use of mechanical implements. Third molars (or "wisdom teeth"), he felt, would be among the next teeth to disappear as the human jaw continued to shrink. As he put it, "As the race becomes more intelligent, the jaw is not required to do so much labor."[5]

Talbot's beliefs about what degeneration of the jaws and teeth meant for an organism as a whole were more complicated. He argued that "from a maxillary and dental stand-point man reached his highest development when his well-developed jaws held twenty temporary and thirty-two permanent teeth. Decrease in the numbers meant, from the dental standpoint, degeneracy, albeit it might mark advance in the man's evolution as a complete being."[6] To illustrate his notion that dental deterioration could serve as a marker of more complete evolution, Talbot offered the example of Americans of African ancestry, to whom he referred frequently throughout his career. "The evolution of the Negro in North America has been most wonderful, mentally and physically," he wrote, "In two hundred and fifty years he has developed from primitive conditions to equal in many cases the Caucasian."[7] Talbot pointed to the gradual recession of black Americans' prognathic tendencies, and their development of flatter and more European-looking facial profiles, as evidence that "the jaw is degenerating for the benefit of the brain."[8]

Talbot speculated that tooth decay and the resultant loss of teeth could best be understood as "natural methods of hastening the process" of man's evolution to a more brain-centered, less tooth-centered organism. As his example

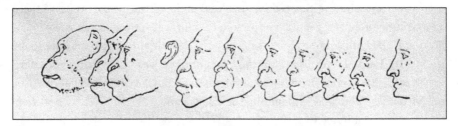

Figure 3 This image placing human profiles in relationship to apes' accompanied Eugene Talbot's description of the dental anatomic changes that occurred during evolution. *Dental Digest* 10 (December 1904): 1.

of the "whitening" of African Americans suggested, he considered this a good thing. In fact, he suggested that it was possible that, although man "from a dental standpoint" had reached his highest state of being when thirty-two healthy teeth were the norm, man as an entire organism might become a higher form of life through the sacrifice of teeth: "A degenerate race," he wrote, "may rank higher in evolution because of the beneficial variations due to degeneracy."[9] Talbot's professional peers concurred in this judgment: "These degenerative changes that we find," mused one commentator in 1902, "are not always for the worst."[10] Using these standards of evaluation, tooth decay could be seen as a positive sign of the progress of evolution in man. Talbot, for one, specifically linked tooth decay with "civilization" more than once. "Notwithstanding all the work that is done for the teeth," he pointed out, "decay is greatly on the increase. It is more common in those who are advanced in civilization and brain development."[11] Several years later, he wrote that "Tooth-decay necessarily goes hand in hand with rise in evolution."[12]

On the other hand, Talbot also believed that tooth decay could be a reliable marker of some of the worst and most deleterious kinds of genetic change—the marker that identified "degenerates" of all stripes. He found "stigmata" of degeneracy, including high levels of tooth decay, among "the idiot, insane, criminal, periodical drunkard, deaf-mute and congenital blind . . . [and] the one-sided genius, the habitual liar, the 'smart' business man, the extreme egotist, the tramp, kleptomaniac, harlot and pauper."[13] Because Talbot thought that the teeth were very sensitive markers of unhealthy degeneracy of the human organism as a whole, he believed that "to alienists, biologists, criminal anthropologists, and sociologists the human jaw and teeth are of peculiar interest, since their study establishes many points in evolution and environment not clearly determinable in other structures."[14] Talbot spent much of his career convincing these other professionals of the importance of teeth as markers for a poor genetic endowment. Later, reflecting on his life's work, he mentioned that he had counseled many prominent European scientists, including Cesar Lombroso, Austrian psychiatrist and sex theorist Richard von Krafft-Ebing, and British physician and sex psychologist Havelock Ellis, both learning from and influencing their ideas about the hereditary nature of crime and sexual vice.[15]

As his reference to "environment" suggested, Talbot's concept of what was inheritable was a fluid one. He felt that inheritable damage could occur through several mechanisms: "ordinary and socially consanguineous marriages, intermixture of races, climate, soil, food, etc."[16] He attributed the most dramatic hereditary damage to nerve weakness in parent or child, which, in turn, could have several discrete causes of its own: among them he listed "excesses involving toxic agents" and "excesses in a social way."[17]

The specific preventive measures Talbot recommended focused almost exclusively on the need to protect one's hereditarily transmissible genetic endowments, or "germ plasm." He recommended against consanguineous marriage (whether "ordinary" or "social"), and against early or late reproduction (before age twenty, or after age forty). He counseled the avoidance of narcotics, alcohol, dangerous occupations, and nervous strain for those of reproductive age. He also warned of the genetic hazards of race-mixing and uncontrolled reproduction, citing a 1652 document's claim that "[in Scotland], if any were visited with the falling sickness, madness, gout, leprosy, or any such dangerous disease which was likely to be propagated from the father to the son, he was instantly gelded; a woman kept from all company of men; and if by chance having some such disease she were found to be with child, she with her brood were buried alive; and this was to be done for the common good, lest the whole nation should be injured or corrupted. A severe doom, you will say, and ought not to be used among Christians, yet more to be looked into than it is."[18] Talbot was a cautious scholar, and it seems possible that his inability to render this advice in his own authorial voice reflected some uncertainty on his part as to either the scientific legitimacy or the social justice of his policy recommendations. The skepticism with which his research and recommendations were received suggests that others shared this uncertainty.

Fellow practitioners challenged the links Talbot attempted to establish between bad teeth and other types of degeneracy. For example, at a 1901 meeting of the American Academy of Dental Science, one dentist suggested that

Talbot had failed to provide an adequate control group of healthy "normal" patients against whom he could compare the dental measurements he took from institutionalized "degenerates," and that Talbot might have misjudged the origin of the poor dental health of those who were under state care. "How would it do," he asked, "to take a comparatively small number of clergymen and measure them very carefully, and, if they presented certain peculiarities, how would it do to conclude that all persons who presented about the same measurements and peculiarities were clergymen?"[19] The absurdity of the suggestion that one could identify clergymen, who acquired their status by dint of long years of dedicated training and scholarship, by the measurements of their teeth, which they acquired through some combination of heredity and environment, highlighted the critic's belief that Talbot had improperly confused qualities which developed through the exercise of human volition and those which were passively acquired. Into this latter category the commentator placed the high rates of tooth decay among the incarcerated: "In speaking of the condition of the teeth that Dr. Talbot finds among the insane, I do not think in my experience I have found that the teeth of the insane are in very much worse condition than might possibly be expected from the care which their teeth naturally receive," he wrote. "You must remember that these people take no care of their teeth, and taking into consideration also the kind of food that they have in the public hospitals, what can you expect under such conditions?" he demanded.[20] Finally, he suggested that Talbot's tendency to regard degenerates as irretrievably bad overstated the case: "If you are to decide that a man has certain mental or moral defects because by your measuring instruments he presents certain asymmetries, you naturally decide that it is a defect of evolution and there is nothing to be done for him, and yet the good qualities in that individual may perhaps, as a matter of fact, completely overshadow the bad."[21]

Other contemporaries accepted Talbot's linkage of bad teeth with other manifestations of bad inheritance, and his belief that bad inheritance polluted absolutely, but rejected his proffered solutions to such ills. A Kansas dentist identified as "F.G." Corey suggested that race-mixing was not only not deleterious, but actually had positive effects on both dental and overall physical health. "The nearer kin we marry the nearer to physical wreck we get," he gushed in 1906, "and that is my argument that the new blood or foreign blood is what is saving our people physically, but it does seem a pity, to have to commingle with some foreigners, but we must remember that we are all the offspring of foreigners."[22] Corey chastised the members of ethnic groups known for their reproductive insularity, especially Germans and Jews, and gave recommendations for race mixtures that were likely to be particularly successful: "The Iberic or Spanish people make a good cross with the people in Southern United States, also the Semitic, the Jew especially," he said.[23] Corey contradicted contemporary fears about the impact of white Americans' "race suicide," arguing that better Americans were to be had from race mixture than from any other kind of reproduction. "We have always called that American Indian the true American," he mused, "but today I have another true American, the Indian, Irish, Scotch, Iberic, Semitic, and all of their descendants crossed. What could make a stronger race than a true American from so many strains of blood?"[24]

Like others of his time, Corey believed that reproduction ought to be carefully, perhaps even legally, controlled; he just differed dramatically in his opinion of the ways in which that control ought to be exercised. "If we could control or educate our children as to what kind of people they should marry to better their children's condition, I think it would be a practical thing to do," he said. "In this way we could get any kind of beauty we might desire, any kind of teeth we might require, and the strongest upon the earth."[25] Corey's association of beauty, good dental health, and the progress of civilization differed from Talbot's insistence that tooth decay could actually be a sign of good evolutionary progress. This alone, suggesting as it did that the 90 percent of Americans who suffered tooth decay didn't just have degenerating teeth, but were actually degenerates, might have been seen as radical—especially while persuading immigrants to become more like Americans remained so high on the national agenda. It was clear however that Corey expected his revolutionary ideas about race and reproduction to engender the most dramatic resistance: perhaps they already had. Near the end of one public talk on the subject, he warned that "no foolish correspondence will be answered, as I have taken up this theme only for pastime and not to lose my life."[26]

The audience at Corey's talk did not embrace his theory of race and reproduction, though they did accept his association of good teeth with good health. Another of the attendees at Corey's lecture opined that "It is our duty to preserve all the teeth possible; to develop the jaw by service and the younger portion of the present generation will have the teeth so set in the arch so that the contour and perfect formation of the arch will be preserved, and a better physical condition will be the result, without any crossing with some of the other races."[27] Talbot, convinced that dental degeneration and higher brain development often occurred together, might have regarded this dentist's admonition to "preserve all the teeth possible" as regressive. It was far more common for dentists to view good teeth as a marker of overall well-being.

Early twentieth-century dentists' ideas about the role of inheritance in producing bad dental health were complicated almost to the point of incoherence. Contemporary thinkers about the role of genetics in dental health differed in their evaluation of the meaning of good (or bad) dental health, the question of whether good dental health ought to be sought after, the means by which it could be attained, and their beliefs about who ought to make such decisions. This muddled intellectual context prevented dentists from enthusiastically concluding that an individual's genetic makeup fixed his or her prospects for dental health for life. Instead, a prevailing spirit of enthusiasm about the likelihood of successful health interventions, spurred in part by the research successes of bacteriologists and the warm reception given to pilot dental hygiene programs, provided a platform for a different theory of dental decay. This school of thought looked to controllable diet rather than to uncontrollable inheritance to explain where bad teeth came from. Like Talbot's and Corey's differing ideas about heredity, the early twentieth-century arguments over diet provided a forum for multiple opinions about meaning, causation, and responsibility. At its peak, the argument that diet controlled dental health also gave rise to one of the most powerful and radical critiques of American culture and politics to emerge from the health professions before the middle of the century.

Tooth Decay as a Product of Diet

Scientific thought about eating changed dramatically in the early decades of the twentieth century. Dentists in this period worked in the shadow of the "New Nutrition," an invention of home economists who had reacted to the discovery of protein, fats, and carbohydrates by creating meals intended to provide an ideal balance of the three. The home economists' interest in promoting themselves as the practitioners of a scientific trade led them to ignore taste and texture beyond the minimum attention necessary to produce meals acceptable to American habits of the table.[28] Standardization, more than any other characteristic, exemplified the changes in Americans' diets in the first half of the twentieth century. New technologies in canning, packing, and hybridization, including the 1903 invention of the virtually indestructible iceberg lettuce, had made American eating habits portable across state—and class—lines. Delicacies, like salads, that had once been available only to the wealthy few were increasingly to be seen on the tables of the bourgeois as well.[29] Americans were, as food historian Harvey Levenstein puts it, "liberated from seasonality [by] improvements in transportation, preservation and distribution. . . . The shelves of an A&P in Louisville, Kentucky, were hardly distinguishable from the shelves of one in Utica, New York, or Sacramento, California."[30]

Even the renowned nutritional rebels of the day were not immune to the logic of dietary standardization, or to the home economists' blithe unconcern for the palatability of healthful food. Turn-of-the-century American nutritional faddist Horace Fletcher advocated chewing each mouthful of food no less than one hundred times, "until it had absolutely no taste and was involuntarily swallowed."[31] Vegetarian John Harvey Kellogg, whose Battle Creek, Michigan, company was to make its meat-replacing breakfast cereals a standard on American tables within twenty years, shared Fletcher's belief that "the decline of a nation commences when gourmandizing begins." A nutritionist at the fourth conference of the American Home Economics Association lamented similarly in 1904 that "local tastes and family idiosyncrasies" still exerted a powerful influence over the dinner table, preventing the development of "conscious standards" in meal planning. "The 'breaking of bread' is a universal sacrament and it is given to men primarily for the strengthening of their bodies, not for the gratification of their palates. To make the choice of food a matter of whims and unreasoning habit . . .—is this not to forget the first law of social righteousness, 'Man shall not live unto himself alone'?"[32]

The combination of scientific and moral urgings toward dietary conformity, and the technological advances making such conformity possible, extended into social workers' attempts to Americanize the diets of the poor. In the view of the leaders of this newly professionalized discipline, the only trouble with the national standardization of eating habits was that it had not progressed far enough down the economic ladder.[33] Home economists promoted dietary standardization as a means of mitigating the criminal and revolutionary tendencies of some immigrant groups, particularly Italians, Jews, and Mexicans.[34] The combined efforts of social workers and advertisers, together with the assimilative pressure of the public schools and the military, were widely successful in enforcing dietary conformity on all but Southern Italian immigrants, whose native cuisines survived these forces more or less intact.[35]

Physicians and home economists were particularly interested in standardizing the diets of infants. Shocked at the high rates of infant mortality in the late nineteenth century, physicians had begun as early as the 1890s to recommend formula or, in an earlier incarnation, "percentage" feeding to mothers whose children failed to thrive on breast milk.[36] While they recognized that the death rate for bottle-fed infants was actually higher than that for breast-fed ones, physicians argued that this was because the living conditions of bottle-fed infants of the time were frequently so much worse than that of children who were breast-fed: in concert with social work, they believed, science could solve these problems, too. Thus, physicians wary of the nervous exhaustion of new mothers and of the moral qualifications of wet nurses increasingly recommended that women unable or unwilling to nurse their infants consider bottle feeding as a healthful alternative. Throughout the 1920s, physicians struggled for dominance with manufacturers of patent infant foods, who had taken to printing such clear instructions for use on their packages that mothers could formula-feed their infants without medical advice.[37] Advocates of "scientific motherhood" argued that women's maternal instincts needed to be generously supplemented with medical expertise in order to ensure the health of children.[38] "Modern" mothers chose bottle feeding, frequently under pressure from physicians, increasingly throughout this period.

During this period of anxious focus on the standardization of the American diet, scientists and the American public became virtually obsessed with vitamins. Contemporaneous with the discovery of these chemical substances was the mass delusion that even Americans with calorically adequate diets were usually not getting enough of them. Nutritionists and physicians argued that ignorance and poverty led many Americans to make poor food choices; even those who did choose correctly often destroyed the vitamin content of what they ate through "modern" food processing techniques.[39]

Though everyone seemed to agree that a more standardized American diet would be a positive change, there was much disagreement about who ought to set the standards for that diet. In fact, the widespread belief that one right way to eat would eventually be divined seemed to heighten the tension between and among professionals about whose job it would be to do it. In 1905, for example, one dentist told the Odontographic Society of Chicago that "Diet is certainly a very important and practical subject, one, it seems to me, that we should discuss more frequently than we do in our meetings."[40] At the same meeting, another dentist closed the comment period by pointing out that "We have had the pleasure this evening of listening to a paper which some years ago might have been pronounced out of accord with our character of work, and yet it is being recognized every day that the subject of dietetics is an important part of our curriculum and work.'[41] The speaker's use of the passive voice ("might have been pronounced") makes it difficult to discern precisely who it was who might have done that pronouncing—dentists themselves? Nutritionists? Physicians? Patients?

Dentists faced opposition from all four groups in their attempts to stake a claim to professional expertise about diet. Like late nineteenth-century public health officials who had moved slowly toward regulation of the food supply, dentists were reluctant to sully their tenuous reputations for scientific authority by venturing into an area in which the state of the art was so freshly developed. Food purity was generally understood as the province of moral reformers rather than researchers.[42] As with other moral reform movements, some of the most vigorous advocates of dentists' participation in dietary reform were women, whose scarcity in the profession reflected their perceived lack of scientific capacity—and therefore, the lack of scientific authority associated with positions they took. Dentists who advocated dietary change had to expound the message to their peers repeatedly before it stuck. One practitioner noted of a meeting of the Odontographic Society of Chicago that "a large number of the dentists present, whom I met before the meeting, felt that [diet] was scarcely a subject that pertains to dentistry, but the discussion this evening has conclusively proven, if it has proven any one thing, that it is primarily a dental subject."[43] Some dentists needed quite a bit of prodding on this score. In 1919, one article on diet republished in a prominent dental journal was preceded with an editorial note: "Is it not about time that YOU showed some interest in this matter?—Editor."[44] Despite more than twenty years of commentary on the relationships between teeth and food, in 1922 pedodontist M. Evangeline Jordon, who wrote extensively about nutrition and dental health in the 1920s and 1930s, was still trying to convince her fellows at an American Dental Association meeting that "the signs of the times clearly point to the fact that the dentists of the country must organize [around the subject of diet], for the care of the teeth of the pre-school child or lose their professional standing."[45]

Pediatricians viewed dentists' interests in diet as illegitimate incursions into their own professional turf, and resisted dentists' attempts to prescribe diets to young patients. During the discussion of Jordon's ADA paper, a Portland, Oregon, dentist pointed out that one pediatrician attending the convention had argued in his own presentation that "Dentists have no right to interfere in the selection of a child's diet."[46] Another discussant explicitly framed the conflict as one of dentists' own right to professional respect: "We know that diet is the greatest factor in caries," he said, "And it does not seem to be consistent with our professional degree, that we should not be allowed to prescribe diet."[47] A final questioner asked Jordon herself to comment on the proper limits of the dentists' authority, entertaining a possibility that no doubt struck audience members as radical: "To what extent is the dentist . . . warranted in prescribing diet in case we find the pediatrician or general practitioner is not giving a proper diet according to our viewpoint? Are we warranted in removing the case from their hands, if possible, or advising the removal and change to another pediatrician or another practitioner?"[48] Pediatricians' seeming primacy in matters of childhood diet prevented more dentists from embracing the subject as part of their own professional domain—but some dentists, at least, were not ready to knuckle under to pediatricians' pressure.

The American public apparently also needed persuasion that their dentists were appropriate sources of good nutritional advice—or, at least, dentists thought they did. In this task, again, dentists frequently conceded the feminization of concern for nutrition by having women characters and narrators deliver nutritional advice. In 1922, for example, the *Dental Digest* published a series of propaganda pieces for subscribers to submit to their local newspapers as part of ongoing efforts to raise the visibility and status of the dental profession. "A Dentist's Wife and His Health" acknowledged that the public was more ready to accept input on diet from the women associated with dentists than from dentists themselves. Written in the voice of the dentist's wife, the article described her phone conversation with "Mrs. So and So," who was concerned about her own run-down husband and had called on the telephone to find out what the dentist ate. The dentist's wife told "Mrs. So and So" that her husband ate lightly, drank no tea or coffee, smoked "very little," and "loves to be out of doors as much as possible." This was all a change, she observed, from when they were first married, and the dentist's poor diet made him nervous, irritable, and less productive than he could have been otherwise. The dentist's rejuvenation was a personal triumph for both husband and wife: the article concluded with the news that "Several months ago he was 'looked over' by a physician and had his teeth X-rayed. The physician told him in medical terms that he had nothing the matter with him. . . . Today if you happen to meet him and ask him how he felt he would answer, 'Fine. Couldn't feel better,' or an equivalent for those words."[49] The item, part of a "public education" campaign to "inform the public of the possible results of dental ignorance or neglect," sought to persuade its skeptical readers that their dentists (and their dentists' wives) were likely to have special dietary knowledge that patients ought to seek out.[50]

Dentists' earliest attempts to establish links between diet and dental decay saw them turning to the well of comparison for evidence: international travel in connection with military service, missionary work, and the vacationing in which dentists of rising affluence frequently engaged forced them to observe the generally good dental health of the people in the places they visited. Multiple observers pointed to the need for the kind of expert technical dental care in which American dentists increasingly took pride as prima facie evidence that there was something deeply, and uniquely, wrong with Americans' teeth—and perhaps with America itself. In 1901, for example, when dentists at the meeting of the Northeastern Dental Association discussed a presentation on "Nutrition as a Tooth-Builder," one Worcester, Massachusetts, dentist rose to point out that "In Calcutta there are only two dentists to-day." He interpreted the low priority that Indians placed on dentistry as evidence of their abundant good health rather than of their disregard for scientific progress: he added that "They have no occasion for dentists, and, as I understand it, this is their simple argument for a grain diet as tooth-builders . . . I believe in one day's time I saw more perfect teeth than in thirty years of practice. It speaks something, certainly, for the practice of grain diet."[51] The nutritional bankruptcy of the American diet, some writers observed, was contagious: in 1902, speaking at another meeting of the Northeastern Dental Association, Boston dentist Gustave Wiksell objected to the notion that there was something about the extremes of the American climate that caused teeth to decay, pointing out that "if it is our climate, how do we explain that before American-process flour was shipped to Sweden, two generations ago, two dentists were enough for the whole city of Stockholm, whereas now they are as thick as in an American city? My friends, God cannot make a four-year-old colt in four minutes, nor can He make teeth out of starch."[52]

Americans had come to believe that describing something as "American" implied praise, not condemnation. Indeed, with their campaigns to increase the level of education and training required for entry to their profession, and with the Progressive-era vigor that characterized their hygiene programs, American dentists themselves played a critical role in establishing the legitimacy of such a connection as it applied to dental care. Therefore, the idea that there was something unusual about Americans' eating habits, and that it was that unique Americanness that caused dental decay and ill health, required constant reinforcement; Americans frequently lost track of the notion when emphasis shifted elsewhere. Throughout the early twentieth century, dentists explicitly linked nationality and national eating habits with dental health status. As early as 1898, for example, one New Hampshire dentist argued that "Perhaps among no other people are dental lesions greater than with the English-speaking races . . . but of the peasantry of Europe there seems good ground for the opinion that they possess better teeth than the poorer people of America."[53] Pointing to the growing number of "lunatics, drunkards, criminals· and epileptics"[54] in the United States, dentists found explanation for their numbers in the knowledge that "In no land under the sun is there such utter disregard of the standing resolutions of good health in regard to diet as in the United States."[55]

Perhaps this repetition was necessary because dentists themselves had not come to a unanimous conclusion about the meaning of the term "American" with respect to the quality of food products or of diets more generally. Their attempts to assign a nationality to the problem of food adulteration epitomized dentists' confusion on this point. Dentists imagined themselves as part of a national surveillance apparatus directed at the food industry: "We should see that foods are stamped with the names of their ingredients," one dentist wrote in 1901, "and those which are adulterated and unfit for food should be avoided and the sellers brought before the law and punished for their crime—for I consider adulteration of foods nothing less than a crime."[56] The 1906 Pure Food and Drug Act mandated the accurate labeling of foodstuffs and made many commonly used food additives (like preservatives, coloring, or flavoring) illegal. Both before and after the passage of the act, the addition of harmful chemicals to otherwise wholesome food proved a persistent concern. One story, reprinted in several nationally distributed dental journals in 1921, described "A Chemist's Adventure in 'Jam,'" in which a curious chemist discovered that a jar of "strawberry" jam actually consisted of an apple base blended with artificial color and strawberry flavor. Puzzled by the jam manufacturer's ability to create lifelike strawberry "seeds," he took his wife's suggestion to plant the seeds and "see what comes up," only to discover that he "got a fine crop of clover!"[57]

Some dentists described food adulteration as one of the principal flaws of the American diet, complaining that doctoring bread with sawdust, flour with talc, and foods of all kinds with potentially toxic preservatives was so common in the United States that it had come to be practically pathognomic of the American way of eating—and, indeed, of the American way of living. "There seems scarcely a product that has escaped," wrote A. B. Spach in

1905, "A cause of the much-talked-of race suicide can be found here."[58] But, depending upon the prevailing political winds, dentists also constructed the adulteration of food as a quintessential un- (or even anti-) American problem, as illustrated by a 1918 filler piece exhorting dentists to do their part for national defense, and referencing the Germans' reported wartime practice of using wood-derived cellulose fibers instead of flour as a basis for bread-making. "If we don't want wooden bread, paper shoes, tin money, perpetual militarism, systematic german atrocities in business, german 'kultur,' and a german substitute for civilization, we've got to win this war!" it proclaimed.[59] Peacetime complaints about the flaws of the American system sometimes evanesced under the pressure of war. There was, however, a persistent thread of concern about the American diet, and its effects on other aspects of American life, in dentists' professional conversations.

The other particulars of dentists' complaints about Americans' eating habits fell into several categories. The most often repeated was a concern about the nutritional impoverishment of white "American-process" flour, which had had the fibrous bran stripped from it, and which was increasingly used not only in home baking but in store-bought breads and pastries.[60] The latter often merited a separate mention as items of particularly pernicious influence. "White flour is adulterated food," one dentist argued in 1901.[61] Gustave Wiksell indulged in a vivid screed against white flour in 1902: "Abolish flouring mills and you will abolish dentistry and all nerve troubles," he proclaimed, "Gunpowder is less dangerous in the house than fine flour. . . . Let me make the bread of the people, and I care not who makes the pills!"[62] Though one of Wiksell's colleagues rose to chide him for his extremism on the issue of white flour ("I cannot think all of the sins of this earth to-day should be laid upon the shoulders of those who grind flour," a man identified as "Dr. Barrett" griped[63]), and though other practitioners occasionally dissented from the popular disdain of white flour, Wiksell had many allies in his professional suspicion of the product. Even "Dr. Barrett's" crotchety objections to anti-flour extremism seem to have been more to radicalism in general than to the disparagement of white flour itself: he also mocked nutritional reformer Alexander Graham, whose "very elaborate and astonishing theories concerning vegetarianism and unbolted flour have been the asylum and sanctuary for every eccentric and extremist and reforming radical from the day in which he wrote his first pronunciamento down to the present time, and have probably saved the infliction upon us of many a crude and undigested theory by the long-haired men and short-haired women who have found satisfaction and rest as 'Grahamites.'"[64] In 1912, a dentist reported to the Maryland State Dental Association that one of his patients had developed enormous cavities in his previously healthy teeth after eating bread from his own bakery, despite having taken meticulous care of his teeth. This prompted the dentist to study the connection between white bread and dental decay further. He discovered "caries quite prevalent among the . . . individuals who ate bakers' bread exclusively."[65]

Like the consumption of refined flour, excessive consumption of refined sugar also disturbed dentists. They posited several mechanisms by which sugar could damage the teeth: one practitioner reported that Americans' sugar consumption led to the creation of excess stomach acid, which traveled up to the teeth and caused them to decay—an affliction known in Europe as "the Yankee disease."[66] A 1922 survey of American dentists found thirteen of fourteen agreeing that candy was bad for the teeth and should not be sold to children, though they differed about the means by which candy's sugar content did its damage.[67] The lack of clarity regarding sugar's effects on teeth, and the mechanism thereof, gave rise to several novel plans for studying the question: a Chicago dentist suggested that diabetics be used as a control group. By the mid-1920s, common wisdom more frequently referenced Americans' sugar habit as a cause of poor dental health. "I find the greatest offense against the laws of dietetics is the feeding of too much sugar," M. Evangeline Jordon wrote in 1923.[68] Slowly, practitioners came to the conclusion that excess sugar, even in an otherwise balanced diet, could be profoundly injurious: "Often when milk desserts are made," complained one dietician who spoke at a dental society meeting in the same year, "they are so sweet that much of the nutritional value is counteracted by the effects of the all too prevalent American high sugar diet."[69] Another complained that schools' insistence on selling candy to children undermined the food habits teachers and dentists were trying to teach those children: "Eating candy," he opined, "is a characteristically American habit, that is formed early in life."[70]

Meat also preoccupied American dentists; its consumption seemed to some to be among the most injurious of American dietary habits. Some early twentieth-century dentists advocated vegetarianism, agreeing with John Harvey Kellogg that meat products were difficult to digest and prone to fermentation in the human intestinal tract, causing disease. "Flesh, together with other indigestible foods . . . [are] the greatest causes of indigestion, which nine-tenths of the American people are afflicted with to-day. Indigestion is one of the greatest causes of constitutional deterioration, resulting in the

decay and loss of teeth," argued an Ohio dentist, who believed that the structure of human teeth suggested that "man is not carnivorous by nature . . .
man's mouth and teeth are a mill," best suited for grinding grain products and
vegetable foods.[71] An Arizona dentist advised readers of *Oral Hygiene* that he
would choose foods "from the fruit and vegetable class and leave out all the
animal products as immoral, unclean and disease-producing."[72] Meat's contribution to poor digestion—and thereby, in the contemporary understanding, to disgruntledness and criminality—may have been on his mind when
he described it as "immoral." On the other hand, the editor's introduction
to the article suggests that readers might have been expected to connect the
author's disdain for meat with other social and environmental causes of the
day: "Dr. Teufert has made an exhaustive study of diet and has come to practically the same conclusions reached by Upton Sinclair, Hereward Carrington
and hosts of others," the editor wrote. "There is meat in his paper, if not in his
diet."[73] *Oral Hygiene*'s editors were particularly meat-averse: at the end of a
case report of a man who had swallowed his denture plate while eating meat,
suffered "coughing and expectoration of foul smelling pus" for two years,
submitted to two unsuccessful operative attempts to remove the plate (which
was "lodged in his oesophagus at the bifurcation of the trachea"), and finally
died, the author of the report advised that patients with partial plates ought
to be warned of those items' dangers. The editor quipped: "Why not make the
moral, don't eat meat?"[74]

Some dentists, however, recoiled at the thought of a meatless diet.
Another *Oral Hygiene* article reported that though Ralph Waldo Emerson was
said to have avoided meat in the interests of his poetry, the haler and heartier
evolutionist Herbert Spencer reportedly "lived for six months upon this [veg-
etarian] diet, [and] threw everything he had written during this period into
the fire."[75] A Chicago dentist smugly said that that he knew a dentist who
had tried a vegetarian diet: "He is reported to have made many a meal upon
watermelon. . . . He died last winter from tuberculosis."[76] Ultimately, most
dentists rejected vegetarianism, but counseled moderation in the consumption of meat.

Dentists objected to the intake of too much meat or too much sugar, but
some were of the opinion that the real problem with the American diet was
simply that it provided too much food. These dentists believed that high-
calorie diets, like those including meat, were suited only to those who required
large amounts of excess energy, which "city dwellers" did not. "The habits of
eating that a farmer can indulge in are not permissible to the bookkeeper or

salesgirl," one writer warned.[77] Meat, as a particularly concentrated food, was to be avoided not for its inherent defects but simply because it represented too much of a good thing. "We, as American people, are too great eaters," another dentist observed, "We eat too much." He speculated that "Our diet is going to change materially during the next twenty-five years."[78] In wartime, overeating was described by one commentator as "the Real American Peril": "The American dinner table is the most tempting in the world," he sighed in 1918, "It combines English bounty with French cooking and whereas the Englishman is saved from excess by bad cooking and the Frenchman by small portions, the American has mated the English table and the French cook and the result is joy to his appetite and death to his arteries."[79] One writer construed overeating as a product of both time and political priorities, contributing to the construction of the United States as an exemplar of corrupt modernity: "Gluttony is one of the worst and most pernicious habits of the times," he mused, "Though a difficult thing to do, for the benefit of public health, it may become necessary to adopt a twentieth amendment to the Constitution to regulate the *eating* as well as the *drinking* habit."[80]

Throughout the early twentieth century, dentists pointed to the social and scientific energy directed toward modern agriculture as a model to be followed by Americans in pursuit of healthy teeth. These practitioners were disgusted by the disjuncture between Americans' attentiveness to their crops and livestock and their inattention to their dental health. In 1905, an Illinois dentist criticized farmers for limiting the quantity and types of food available to their driving horses, but failing to exercise similar caution about the foods they allowed their children to consume.[81] The example of the stock animal was widely used by dentists who may have been only very recently off the farm themselves, though they were careful to explain agricultural references for the benefit of those of urban lineage: "The progressive live stock breeder, who wishes to produce in his young animal the greatest growth of muscle, bone and constitution, feeds them middlings," one dentist commented in 1905.[82] He went on to define "middlings" ("the parts of the wheat which we discard in making our flour"[83]).

The increasing participation of government in agriculture and urban services in the early twentieth century outraged dentists who professed to view human beings as more valuable resources than livestock or real estate. Like the advocates of other contemporary movements for progressive reform, dentists felt that children in particular were entitled to protection from poor food and the dental damage it could cause. "What are the people of the United

States doing to combat [tooth decay] in public schools? Why, nothing! We have plenty of money to fight doodle-bugs, foot and mouth disease among our cattle and infectious disease among hogs, and money for forest preserves," an anonymous writer sputtered in 1911.[84] He went on to describe the exorbitant (in his view) amounts of money that New York City had spent on fire services in one year, asking "Would it not be an economy to spend less money on our cattle and hogs and more on our greatest national asset, the boys and girls of to-day, who are soon to be our rulers and law-makers?"[85] Popular writers echoed this concern, citing the frantic (perhaps, one even suggested, hysterical) efforts to protect crops from invasive insect pests as examples of Americans' misplaced priorities: "In 1919 our agriculturists manifested great alarm lest the European corn borer should spread from the limited regions where it was discovered in New York State and infect other regions where corn is grown," one writer carped in a popular magazine, a portion of which was reprinted in an American dental journal. "The machinery of government was at once set in motion to check the ravages of the European corn borer. Wise indeed is the state that permits itself to be agitated in the presence of the European corn borer. But what about the food deviltries that have been boring unmolested into the health and life of the child?"[86] Dentists viewed the problem of distorted priorities with respect to health and agriculture as a uniquely American one: one writer compared the United States unfavorably with Germany ("a country where they are not only very much concerned about the health of their cattle and hogs, but have the intelligence to look after their school children as well"), Switzerland, and even Russia, where the existence of the St. Petersburg school dental clinic demonstrated Russians' better understanding of the importance of dental health.[87]

As their anger about the misdirection of public resources to animal health and agriculture rather than human health demonstrated, some dentists experienced misgivings about the march of time and the progress of so-called "American civilization," particularly its agricultural—and, relatedly, dietary—manifestations. Eugenicists like Eugene Talbot marked the signs of civilization and eagerly anticipated its furtherance—and were, at times, even willing to sacrifice the health of human teeth and jaws in its service. Others feared that those who lauded the process of civilization had judged wrongly, placing their faith in a way of being that harmed human life more than it enhanced it. One place where this tension played out was in dentists' ongoing debate about the influence of civilization on human appetites and desires. Another was in one prominent dentist's trenchant—but ultimately unsuccessful—critique of American civilization, and particularly of the American diet.

Civilization and Its Discontents

Like other scientists of human heredity, American dentists harbored mixed feelings about the meaning of the term "civilization," and about the effects of civilization on the health of human beings. Charles Darwin and Francis Galton, the preeminent theorists of human heredity, had portrayed civilization as a new cultural development, behind which human nature lagged considerably, and dentists generally shared this view.[88] They frequently contrasted "civilization" with "instinct," as in observations about the difference between a "civilized diet" and the foods to which Americans were drawn to "naturally," by "instinct," or, occasionally, as a result of heeding "appetite." The value judgments implicit in these terms changed dramatically depending on who was using them as reference points.

Some writers used the word "civilization" as a stand-in for qualities that were positive products of social, scientific, and artistic progress. An Ohio dentist argued in 1899 that bad eating habits were a product of unchecked instinct, suggesting that civilization might be a positive restraining force on that instinct: "[T]hat through the depraved, gourmandizing appetite of man, emanating from his debased lower animal nature, his evil habits of life, have their origin I am fully convinced."[89] In this view, the order and purpose imbued in modern life by the trappings of civilization could prove to be a useful corrective to the otherwise injurious whims of the individual. In 1905, dental luminary Frederick Noyes (one of at least three successive generations of dentists in his family) told peers at a meeting of the Odontographic Society of Chicago that "a man who always eats a certain amount, who leaves a clean plate at the end of the meal; always, as a rule, you find that man has lived with comparatively little sickness. On the other hand, a man whose eating is dependent upon his appetite is almost always more or less liable to short periods of sickness, for he will at times overeat, and at other times undereat, and the result is a liability to certain diseased conditions from both causes."[90] That one's own appetite could lead one astray suggested that discipline, in the form of civilized rules for eating, was necessary for good health and long life. This logic helped to make the case for enforcing dietary change on immigrants, whose "instinctive" preferences for their national cuisines was thought to cause poor health, insanity, and political intractability.

On the other hand, many of the Social Darwinists of the turn of the century regarded civilized people's accommodations of the weak—in institutions like public schools, and with measures intended to protect the sick, the poor, or vulnerable recent immigrants—as undesirable interference with the upward progress of human evolution. In this view, too much "civilization" was something to be avoided; "instinct" was to be trusted rather than trained. One Arizona writer admonished his patients to eschew dietary fashion and "use good judgment and be guided by his appetite" when it came to choosing types and quantities of food (though, in case this advice did not suffice, he also gave detailed instructions including the direction to "avoid salt, vinegar, and spices").[91] In these dentists' minds, instinct existed as a permanent subtext of both civilization and savagery, though it had different effects in different conditions. One writer argued that the "preference for the succulent and nutritious" had probably been evolutionarily advantageous for primitive man, since it helped him to supplement an otherwise coarse and bulky diet with more concentrated forms of nutrition.[92] He also seemed to believe that the human capacity to alter food had in fact outstripped the need for that food to be altered—that the mechanical elimination of so much fiber and roughage from the "civilized" diet had redounded in a negative way upon the health status of civilized mankind, and particularly of Americans. "What was at one time performed by the teeth and stomach is now too largely done by machinery and cookery," he wrote, "We may look forward to the time when the food of the uncivilized is correct."[93] In the context of a growing national infrastructure devoted to the production of sweet, sticky, nutritionally bankrupt foods like candy, the instinctive desire to eat soft, sweet things seemed like a hindrance to health rather than a help. Some felt that the dismantling of that infrastructure could restore human instinct to its role as a reliable dining guide.

Most practitioners regarded instinct as a vaguely positive force, though their beliefs about how strong its influence over "civilized" human behavior could (or should) be differed widely. For example, a Copenhagen dentist identified as "Professor Christensen" told a meeting of the International Dental Federation in 1913 that raw carrots were an especially important part of children's diets because they were "pleasant to chew, sufficiently hard while being at the same time brittle enough, so that the child is anxious to overcome the resistance . . . his natural instinct induces him to chew it as small as possible."[94] Chewing, everyone agreed, was a positive good, and any instinct that promoted it would be by definition trustworthy. Yet the presence at the same conference of dietary reformer Horace Fletcher, famed for his insistence that

Americans had to be taught how to chew properly, served as a living example of the proposition that instinct had been all but eliminated by civilization, and that professional guidance was necessary to restore or replace it. This change would take effort, its advocates thought, but it could be done: in his 1923 address to the American Dental Association, the president of that organization urged his listeners to "[have] the courage to change the acquired dietetic habits of the times and recover the lost natural appetite and follow this as their guide."[95]

American dentists never came to a unified conclusion about the relative merits of instinct and civilization. They believed that civilization had led Americans' eating habits astray, but that immigrants' diets should be assimilated to American standards. Outside the context of discussions about the Americanization of immigrants, almost everyone agreed that Americans' diets were bad, but dentists' profound disagreements about whether instinct or civilization would prove a more trustworthy guide to the table gave rise to startlingly divergent analyses of what should be done to improve them. In a notable example of these differences, two women practitioners offered antithetical suggestions as to the merits of allowing young children to make decisions about their own diets. M. Evangeline Jordon commented in 1923 that "the old habit of putting the child at the table in his high-chair, and forgetting or not knowing that children should not eat the same food as their parents, and letting him select his own diet, was followed by so much indigestion and illness that the resistance to disease was greatly lowered and children fell victims to epidemics of measles, scarlet fever, whooping-cough and diphtheria in large numbers. . . . At the present time [health officers' efforts are] being directed toward the forming of *proper habits* in the pre-school age."[96] Jordon believed that children had to be taught to choose what was healthiest for them to eat, and that most dentists and physicians had accepted this reality and advised their patients to abandon the "old habit" of allowing children to choose according to their tastes. Another article published in the same year mourned the fact that not all parents had accepted this dictum wholesale: "Even Grandma humors the child. . . . restriction is needed," pleaded its author. "The child is irresponsible, its powers of judgment are undeveloped and it yields to a well-developed but a perverted taste. . . . [It is] not a question of what the child wants, but what he needs and should have to properly nourish him."[97]

Ironically, despite Jordon's insistence that the instincts of children could not be trusted—and her claim that everyone else accepted this as a fact—one

Cleveland pediatrician would soon embark upon an experiment that seemed to disprove both assertions. In 1926, Clara Davis began what she described as a "self-selection diet experiment in infants and young children" at Mount Sinai Hospital in her home city. Davis directed hospital nurses to offer unlimited quantities of more than twenty different foods to fourteen institutionalized babies at each of their daily meals. The foods were placed in individual bowls, set on high-chair trays, and presented to the infants for their appraisal. Attending nurses were instructed to periodically rearrange the bowls so as to place each of the foods within an infant's easy reach at some point during each meal, but were otherwise "to sit quietly by and not to interfere with anything the baby did. She might not speak to him, call his attention to any food, offer him any or refuse him any for which he reached, comment on what he did or attempt to teach him table manners. Only when he reached for or pointed to a dish was she to take up a spoonful of the food and, if he opened his mouth for it, put it in."[98]

Somewhat to her own surprise, Davis discovered that the instincts of the children in her study led them well. Their eating habits varied wildly, and sometimes disturbingly: Abraham G.'s prolonged "egg jag," culminating in the two-and-a-half-year-old eating ten eggs for supper one night "with no ill effects whatever," particularly unnerved his nurses. But the children grew healthier than they had been on admission to the institution, suffered few common childhood illnesses, and gained weight appropriately—an important measure of child health, particularly among the poor.[99] Davis concluded that "there has existed in [the children] some mechanism made evident as appetite, which, sensitive as a weather vane to every wind that blows, has responded promptly to heat, cold, exercise, fatigue, and infection, and which, when uninterfered with by emotional conflict with elders or suggestions from without, has functioned smoothly and efficiently as far as the simple unmixed foods of this list go."[100] She recommended that parents spend less time and energy "particularizing amounts" of food and coaching their children in eating habits and table manners (though she did concede that parents, like the nurses in her study, might limit the kinds, if not the quantities, of foods to which children had access). These parental—and especially maternal—behaviors, Davis seemed to argue, did harm rather than good to infants' diets and health.

As Jordon's and Davis's differing assessments of instinct—and, by implication, of civilization itself—suggest, these radically opposed opinions could give rise to equally divergent sets of recommendations to parents, patients, and fellow practitioners. If instinct was to be distrusted, and civilization to be regarded as a positive good, then the individual (or the individual's parent or guardian) had a responsibility to ignore instinct and follow the rules of civilization—particularly as handed down by dentists and physicians—as a guide for life. Failure to do so could be interpreted as uncivilized.

Some dentists, like many physicians, considered mothers as technicians in need of constant scientific advice, and regarded the "maternal instinct" as a source of indulgence leading to infection, pain, and ill health. Mothers, in this view, needed help determining not only what to feed their children, but how to feed them. In 1899, dentist Claude Chick chided mothers for their habit, in an age before electric blenders or food processors were available, of pre-chewing their infants' foods. Mothers' ignorance of the harm this practice could cause was an additional strike against them: Chick complained that mothers often claimed not to know what caused their infants' digestive problems, but, he said, "If the physician would examine the teeth of the mother he might get a pointer as to the cause of the trouble. . . . When the mother has several bad teeth broken down by decay, etc., it is very common for her to have pyorrhea, at least her mouth is in a bad state, even for the general health of the mother, leave alone the health of the delicate little child."[101] In 1910, a public-education item used in Rochester, New York, newspapers and reprinted in the *Dental Digest* similarly warned patients and parents against the fate of "Tim," who suffered "numerous stomach disorders . . . generally when his fond mother chewed some delicacy in her own mouth and placed it in his."[102]

Mothers were responsible not only for feeding their children (for good or ill), but for following the rules dictated by science about diet in pregnancy. Some dentists viewed this responsibility as being connected to mothers' responsibility to seek out eugenically sound marriages. Like physicians with interests in eugenics, these dentists promoted the teaching of nutrition, together with sex hygiene curricula, to high school girls, who could not be expected (or allowed) to follow their instinctive preferences in either coupling or eating: "Every girl going through the junior and senior years of high school must have the training in dietetics, especially as applied to prenatal and pre-school feeding, before we will have strong teeth and healthy bodies," predicted one writer in 1923.[103]

On the other hand, if the abrogation of instinct in favor of civilization was a bad thing, then parents, patients, dentists, and government had a whole different set of responsibilities. In fact, if the badness of civilization was itself a cause of dental decay, the deterioration of health, and all other manner of physiological and political ills, perhaps it would take a veritable revolution in Americans' ideas about civilization, and about eating, to reverse the damage caused by progress. The foremost arbiter of this stance in the first half of the twentieth century was a Cleveland dentist named Weston Andrew Valleau Price, the head of the American Dental Association's Research Division and a widely published writer whose works included a classic two-volume text on the links between dental infections and systemic degenerative diseases. Sometime in the 1920s, Price decided to spend much of his spare time traveling around the world to examine the teeth of peoples from a variety of racial and ethnic groups. He believed that his travels could help him to elucidate facts that would be useful for Americans, and for the profession as a whole.

Price, like Eugene Talbot, had begun his career as a vigorous critic of racial miscegenation and its effects on human health. His early writings, including a 1929 talk entitled "Our Children: How We May Add to Or Subtract From their Inheritance," invoked all the standard fears of advocates of eugenic sterilization, including prostitution, sex perversion, and the infamous Jukes family, whose notorious proliferation of ne'er-do-wells was generally regarded as proof of the inherited nature of criminality. Explicitly Lamarckian, Price wrote that "It is by now probably definitely established that it is possible to transmit characters that have been built up by our ancestors. . . . Let's take that terrible picture of the Jukes family. . . . Poorness of those chromosomes was present to this terrible extent that fifty-two percent of the women born in that family [of] twelve hundred individuals were prostitutes, and it is estimated that something over ninety-five to ninety-eight percent of the men were sex perverts."[104] Even as early as 1929, Price expressed some sympathy for the victims of genetic determinism: "They weren't necessarily poor people," he cautioned. "They just had that kind of determiner." But he concluded, like most of his contemporaries, that society had to be protected from the moral and financial consequences of the Jukes' unrestrained reproduction. "Oh, how hard it is," he lamented, "for by law and by restriction we can't eliminate them, to make character. . . . The only way we can do that is to make these people stop producing." In 1929, Price concluded that while government euthanasia campaigns were probably untenable, educational efforts aimed at the marriageable young—as Price put it, "helping to bring God's kingdom on earth"—were not.

Price's world travels turned him from a convinced eugenicist, secure in the belief that human reproduction required scientific help, into the most prominent dietary reformer of his day—a critic of civilization, and a devout believer in the positive power of human instinct. During travels through the South Pacific, he found the locals of many areas possessed of great skill and intelligence when set to work as dentists. In American Samoa, for example, Price gave the natives "pieces of soap and asked them to carve a reproduction of an extracted tooth which was given as a model . . . Their work would probably equal if not exceed in excellence the first effort of 90 per cent of American dental students."[105] More important, though, was what he found when he focused on the dental health of the native peoples of a wide range of locales, most of which were tropical paradises that had been—or were in the process of being—colonized by Western powers. The abundantly good dental health of the locals of virtually everyplace he visited had deteriorated alarmingly after they began eating a Western or "trade" diet—the very same diet that Americans were consuming every day.

By the time he published his magnum opus, *Nutrition and Physical Degeneration*, in 1938, Price had visited isolated groups of "primitive racial stock" on at least four continents. His attentions lingered on the physical condition of non-white natives before and after contact with Westerners. The Samoan islanders were, to Price's eye, finer specimens of humanity than their white colonizers. "The characteristics of the Polynesian race included straight hair, oval features, happy, buoyant dispositions and splendid physiques," he reported.[106] The generations born in Samoa (and elsewhere) after contact with whites suffered from tooth decay, chronic disease, and increased rates of infant mortality. The natives themselves, he suggested, explicitly associated their plight with the presence of whites. He had, as he put it, "found the primitives despising the ignorance of the white man and often endeavoring to shun his influence, by retreating into the jungles or forests. They have observed that the white man's influence is destructive to native tribes."[107] Apparently, the islanders shared some dentists' belief that when health was the measure it was the West, and civilization itself, that suffered in the comparison.

The most common popular explanation for the precipitous decline in both natives' and white colonists' dental health was that race-mixing was to blame. Like other Americans who were regularly exposed by contemporary eugenicists to the notion that the commingling of disparate races could have catastrophic effects, Price had some level of innate sympathy for this explanation, and he investigated it at length. In Fiji, Price reported, the labor demands of sugar plantations resulted in the immigration of large numbers of Indians and Chinese to the island. "This influx of Asiatics together with that of Europeans has had an important influence on the purity of the native race around the ports. This provided an opportunity to study the effects of intermingling of races on the susceptibility to dental caries," he reported, "No differences due to ancestry were disclosed by the presence or absence of tooth decay."[108] Price concluded that the only cause of the skyrocketing rates of tooth decay among natives who engaged in trade and cultural amalgamation with whites was the insufficiency of the white diet. Like the natives themselves, white colonials in the sundry locations Price visited in the early twentieth century seemed to know this, and to feel shame about it. On Thursday Island, north of Australia, Price noted that "an embarrassing situation was encountered with regard to the sensitiveness of the whites in the matter of having their children examined for dental caries."[109] Price and his wife (his constant travel companion, always photographed in seemingly stifling Western dress) had to gauge the dental degeneracy of the colonists there from a distance, by their "irregularities of facial and dental arch development."[110]

Price's discoveries, which convinced him of the singular importance of diet in determining health, permanently changed his feelings about the racist strains of eugenics then in circulation in the United States. Correspondence with his family members suggests the scope and nature of this change. After reading *Nutrition and Physical Degeneration*, which expounded Price's theories on diet and the decay of colonized peoples' health, Price's brother Norman wrote him: "Why so pessimistic? I can't believe mankind is going to the dogs just yet, nor even degenerating so much. The white race is still the most intelligent race; with its engenuity [sic] ways will be found to provide necessary chemicals in our food so we may survive without all living near the sea."[111] Norman Price appealed discreetly to his brother's memory of their shared childhood in rural Ohio: "Do you remember what happened to the boy lambs when we were farm boys? Suggest a law for a similar process in imbeciles."[112] In reply, Price observed that with appropriate nutritional safeguards, both sterilization and euthanasia would be unnecessary.

Nearing the end of his career, Price retained his Lamarckian bent: he believed that the facial deformities and the attendant defects in personality and intelligence caused by poor nutrition might be passed from parent to child, but he also felt that they might be prevented through scrupulous attention to diet on the part of the affected parent. His understanding of heredity was not that much different than Eugene Talbot's: like Talbot, Price thought of heredity as encompassing everything that had an impact on human "germ plasm," including chromosomes, excessive nervous strain, exposure to toxins, and diet. But from this similar conception of heredity, Price developed radically different ideas about "civilization" and its value, suggesting that the political implications of early-twentieth-century ideas about heredity were by no means inevitable.

Modern westerners, Price thought, grew, processed, and ate bad food, and thrust that bad food upon the peoples with whom they came into contact through trade and colonization. The impact of this dietary catastrophe so overwhelmed any other factors influencing human heredity that their significance seemed to pale in comparison. It was the consumption of bad food, not the existence of bad genes, which made the South Sea Islanders seem damaged, incapable of self-care, and in need of the help of white Westerners. In short, Price's analysis was that his contemporaries suffered from the worst sort of observational fallacy. Their presence in unindustrialized areas of the world had caused the illnesses that convinced them that trade and colonization were essential to the "progress" of colonized regions of the globe.

From these facts, one could conclude that the native peoples whom Price studied didn't need white Westerners' help—that the helping relationship, if there was to be one, should flow in quite the opposite direction. Back in the United States, Price sought to convince his colleagues that the evidence of his travels argued strongly for the implementation of "primitive" diets in America. Crowded dental arches and stunted facial growth, he argued, "[had been] wrongly attributed to a mixture of racial bloods" when it was the supplanting of native with white diets that was really at fault.[113]

Price's seemingly simple critique of the dental impact of the modern white diet on previously isolated tribal peoples shrouded his rejection of virtually every major dietary trend of his time. His studies convinced him that diets ought to be carefully chosen to match genetic heritage, which challenged social workers', nutritionists', and physicians' growing belief in the importance of dietary standardization. His observations about the superior health of infants breast-fed by their mothers until one, two or even three years of age ran counter to prevailing wisdom about breastfeeding itself, and to middle-class women's growing use of artificial birth control, rather than extended breastfeeding, as a contraceptive measure. His objection to the use of processed foods challenged the existence of the entire industry; the adoption of his argument for local diets, locally grown, had the potential to undermine the progress made possible by the increasing specialization of modern agriculture. Price considered vitamin supplementation useless, and he posited that vitamin deficiencies originated not in poor foods, but in poor soil.

He advocated organic farming, which posed a threat to both the practice of factory farming and the burgeoning agricultural chemicals industry.

With these other heresies, Price took a vigorous stance in the debate raging in American life about who or what should be held responsible for individuals' health ills and woes. Unlike the pessimists who despaired of changing Americans' dietary habits—and still less their inherited genetic traits—Price believed that American social and economic systems ought to be the target of reformers' outrage, and of focused efforts for change. In this, he opposed those who argued that measures taken at the level of the individual or the household could effectively counteract the damage that might inadvertently be done by the otherwise benevolent systems of capitalism and democracy. Price challenged widespread popular assumptions about the inherent fitness of the American system—the professional, scientific, rational, civilized American system—to be applied to human beings, both domestically and overseas. To Price, the dietary and cultural standardization wrought abroad by colonialism mirrored that which was underway in the United States, and his opposition to one paralleled his opposition to the other. "Surely," he concluded in 1935, "our civilization is on trial both at home and abroad."[114]

Price's research was widely published in the best American dental journals. He had given many years of service and much of great scientific value to the profession before he dared to call into question the wisdom of the American way of life, and his preexisting professional prominence brought him the respect and affection of his professional colleagues, including the journal editors who disseminated his work. Yet his critique of Americans' diets, and of the larger systems of which those diets were a part, barely survived him. After Price's death in January of 1948, his will provided for the republication of *Nutrition and Physical Degeneration*, and a small group of Price's admirers banded together to promote his research findings in other ways. His findings, though, were only rarely mentioned in mainstream professional literature after his death.[115]

In the first half of the twentieth century, dentists increasingly placed the blame for tooth decay, and for many illnesses proceeding from it, squarely on the defects and deficiencies of the modern American way of life. Americans' poor care of their teeth, lamentable habits of uncontrolled reproduction, and flawed dietary predilections each came in for extended criticism by dentists—and, to a certain extent, by other professionals as well. Focus on the volitional causes of poor dental health helped to further the notion that

Americans could—and should—do something to prevent tooth decay, and that it was a positive sign of social and professional progress to do so.

Though their nationalist fervor was challenged by Americans' continued experience of bad dental health, dentists were increasingly convinced that meritorious peoples and nations would share American dentists' concern for the traits of scientific specificity, efficiency, and modernity, all of which American dentists were increasingly coming to see as landmark achievements of the profession. Many dentists, like Weston Price, traveled extensively, and they took careful note of how their professional ideals were received abroad. The other nations in which the United States took interest, these dentists felt, could be assessed and ranked by their esteem for these characteristic features of American dentistry—or by their rejection of them. By the middle of the century, dentists described a high regard for American dental practices as a threshold measure of the value and assimilability of people around the world.

Chapter 3

"Like a Sugar-Coated Pill"

Defining American Dentistry Abroad

In 1921, an author who identified himself as "A Japanese Office Boy" wrote to the editor of *the Dental Digest* to ask a series of impertinent questions about the way Americans practiced dentistry. "Mr. Editor of Small but Helpless Magazine of Toothsome Tendencies," the letter began, "Somewhat Honorable Sir: Recently I have absorbed one complete course, by correspondence, of English decomposition and letter write. . . . Having recently completed all Money Orders, Mr. Editor, I now possess delicious abilities to express thoughts occurring in brains or elsewhere in approximate English and so similarly to all newly arrived Americans I hasten to news print wherever possible. Thank you. Natural comeback for you of Dental Magazine Editorship is 'Why pick on me?'" The author, who also referred to himself as "Houseboy," explained that his most recent jobs had been in dentists' offices, and that he was confused about what he had witnessed there. For example: "Why will ambidextrous tooth tormentor insist on placing Dams composed of rubber and profane language over helpless teeth when cotton rolls of entire whiteness will accomplish same purpose in many cases in 1/8 elapsed time while also allowing chair victims to completely retain all Christian expressions formerly used during operations of open faced nature? Answers should be tabulated when convenient." The letter was signed "Yours if necessary, TOGO."[1]

The article appeared below an editorial note admonishing: "Even if this hits you (which it is quite apt to do) you will like it. Like a sugar-coated pill it will do you good—pleasantly—(Editor.)"[2] The satire of "Togo's" letter embodied the animus of its white author, and many of his race and social class, toward the perceived infiltration of American public spaces by immigrants. Within three years of the publication of "Togo's" missive, American immigration law, already restrictive with respect to Asians, would be revised so as to effectively exclude all Asian immigration to the United States. The "letter," therefore, cannot be understood apart from the history of increasing anti-Asian nativism in the United States in the 1920s.

The document had a function beyond political commentary, though: it parroted the voice of an immigrant who had no business offering a critique of the United States or its dental practices in order to goad American dentists into better behavior. Lacking formal education, English fluency, and wisdom, even "Togo" could see that some American dentists' practices made no sense. "Togo's" letter was funny not only because of its garbled English, but because it inverted the social conventions of early twentieth-century American professional racism, and upended the conventions of a genre with which American dentists were extremely familiar: the dental travel essay.

In the first few decades of the twentieth century, as the sectional tension of the mid- to late nineteenth century gave way to the nationalist excursions of the Spanish-American War and World War I, American dentists traveled for military and missionary work that sought to spread the gospel, the arm of the Republic, and an improved standard of dental treatment far and wide. Their commitment to the political and military context for their journeys meant that most dentists, unlike Weston Price, were proud of the qualities they associated with Americanness; their travels caused them to more tightly connect professional behavior with a positive national identity.

Dental travelers produced an enormous volume of writing describing their experiences abroad and the conditions of dental practice in the places they visited. They hoped to edify, to entertain, and to agitate their peers with their writings. In so doing, they also imbued the term "American dentistry" with specific meaning. The metropolitan American identity to which they appealed was constructed in part by their surveillance and characterization of American peripheries—often, locations that had been colonized by the United States.[3] An important effect of the travel writing published in dental journals in this period was to define what people, and what dental and societal practices, could rightfully be denominated "American," particularly as calibrated against people and practices that would fail of this aspiration. Consistency, sophistication, specificity of diagnoses, remedies, and procedures, firm but fair licensing laws, temperate climates, efficiency in billing

and paying, cleanliness, promptness, commitment to meritocracy, and interest in appearance were American: their antagonists were not.

Of course, these qualities were not consistently present in the United
States, or in dentists who practiced there. The authors of dental travel essays
emphasized such traits partly because their existence in the United States
was so uncertain—and, at times, so bitterly contested. Yet dental travel writing, like other professional and popular discourse at home, militated toward
those attributes, and toward their cultivation in places abroad that came
under American purview. It thus contributed equally to burgeoning concepts
of what was "professional" in American dentistry. Eventually, description
and discussion of dental practice in areas occupied, annexed, or merely contemplated by the United States helped to inform discussions about what relationship the United States ought to have to those locations, and about how
successful such connections were likely to be.

The Role of Dental Journals and Dental Travel Writing

Early twentieth-century dentists eager to shape themselves to dentistry's rising professional standards welcomed dental journals into their mailboxes as
valuable sources of information and guidance. Though dentists were sepa-
rated from one another by their varying levels of education and aspiration,
as well as by geographic distance and the resultant shortage of opportunities
for communication in real time (like attending conferences, or even speaking to one other on the telephone), journal reading and writing helped to
create an imagined community of practitioners who increasingly shared a
professional identity as American dentists.[4] Journals contained articles
describing the most basic of dental procedures in great detail, for the benefit
of those who were trying to teach themselves new techniques without the aid
of either schools or fellow dentists. Frequently, journals would reprint the
entire proceedings of especially noteworthy conferences, including complete
transcripts of question-and-answer periods after scholarly papers. They also
offered direct advice about office procedures and relationships with patients.
Journals worked to create a shared identity for dentists by making remarks
on national and international political concerns, providing descriptions of
appropriate "professional" behavior around patients, and periodically inter-
jecting classical literary and artistic references, carefully but not condescend-
ingly explained to the reader who lacked a liberal education.

The journals provided education and mutual uplift, and created a community of insiders that would constitute a profession: dental travel writing

helped to accomplish all of these ends. The missteps of ill-informed dentists abroad taught lessons about what was expected of dentists at home. For the writer and the reader, travel writing had the special benefit of working to raise the shared standard of professionalism without acknowledging the wide divergence of conditions then prevailing in domestic dentists' offices. Direct reference to the fact that, for example, some American dentists failed to sterilize their instruments was unnecessary when a writer could point to the same omission by a foreign dentist, and then link foreignness with lack of hygiene, unscientific practice, and poor professional judgment to make the same point.

Published dental travel writing sought to enhance the cosmopolitanism of American dentists, who could not be assumed to have acquired either a comprehensive formal education or an international outlook. For example, in 1927, the dental journal *Oral Hygiene* published a series of articles by D. T. Parkinson, a Wichita dentist then engaged as a teacher and practitioner on a round-the-world trip with a "University Afloat." Parkinson advised readers that the trip was intended to "[add] to the usual curriculum of the school the advantages of world travel": the articles themselves were intended to do the same for American dentists, and Parkinson saw no need to explain what "the advantages of world travel" might be.[5] Many of the American elite aspired to a period of European travel before entering a profession, and journals tended to assume the prevalence of this standard—and, discreetly, to provide remedial education for readers whose own experience had fallen short of the norm. As a result, American dental journals occasionally ran travel narratives whose sole purpose was diversion—these mentioned local dental practices fleetingly, if at all, and often in ways that suggested that such practices had been observed from a touristy distance rather than from the professional point of view. Such articles appeared less frequently as standards of education and licensing in the United States increased, and as the doors of practice were slowly but firmly closed to those who lacked comprehensive undergraduate education and its associated bourgeois tastes, including the taste for foreign travel.

The authors of dental travelogues admired the teeth of the native peoples in the places they visited. They also generally shared Eugene Talbot's belief that excellent dental health signified delayed progress up the ladder of evolution, and that it was usually accompanied by an unseemly disregard for the importance of civilization. Together with the advocates of public dental hygiene programs and the dietary reformers who lauded civilization over instinct, they took the position that whatever excess of dental defects Americans suffered as a result of their advancement through the stages of civilization could be remedied with uniquely American applications of dental training and ingenuity. This, they felt, was a sign of the superiority of the United States and of the American way of life.

Dental travelogues implying or directly stating this most commonly came from American writers, but American dental journals also regularly published missives sent by British and other English-speaking correspondents. Whatever the nationality of their authors, such items focused almost exclusively on the question of how indigenous peoples' dental health and dental practices compared with those of Americans. The priority that American journals placed on publishing these items suggests that the editors of these journals—and, perhaps, their readers—saw this international agreement as an important confirmation of their own assessment of the matter.

Conquest, Conversion, and Dentistry

Most American dental travelers were connected, either formally or informally, to the US military. Army dentists reported from outposts in Cuba, the Philippines, Puerto Rico, and Hawai'i in the early twentieth century—all had been acquired, with greater or lesser degrees of formal connection, by the United States as a result of the 1898 Spanish-American War.[6] By mid-century, reports emanated from the Soviet Union, Japan, China, and some locations in Africa as well. Military dental practitioners provided valuable service to American servicemen and their dependents, who might have been unable to obtain satisfactory dental treatment otherwise: "The dental officer of the navy . . . is the only dentist in American Samoa," Lieutenant Commander H. J. LaSalle reported in 1933.[7] American dentists also treated the native peoples in the places they visited, and were viewed as important contributors to the project of pacifying the locals in many regions. The military governors of such locations saw the importance of having reputable dental care available: legislation signed by the military governor of the Philippines as early as 1907 required the nation's dental board to license three dentists who had graduated from accredited dental schools in the United States. The dentist who reported this observed that "when the first expedition was sent to the islands, the necessity of protecting the soldiers from empirical practitioners and quacks was recognized."[8]

Often following close behind military dentists were dental travelers who worked as missionaries. They, too, believed that the ability to practice

high-quality dentistry upon indigenous populations and on fellow evange-
lists was of critical importance. In 1921, the *Dental Digest* reported that "One
of the first jobs of the American missionaries among the Awembi in Central
Africa is to handle the dental forceps . . . one of the best preparations for
successful missionary work is a good dental course, and one very useful gift
which can be bestowed upon the man departing for a foreign field is a well-
equipped case of dental supplies."[9] The *Digest*, which headlined the item
"Winning Souls Through the Dental Forceps," observed that dental care was
an important facet of a successful proselytization program: "The man who
is not armed with modern dental supplies has his chance of winning souls
lessened," it claimed.[10]

Dental missionaries wrote enthusiastically of the importance of dental
work partly because they had difficulty persuading the religious sponsors of
missions of it. This difficulty reflected the resistance to dental care faced by
practitioners in the United States from their stateside patients, among whom
were the church leaders responsible for setting priorities in missionary work.
At times, missionaries complained frankly that dental work was the most
neglected aspect of evangelism. From India, one missionary wrote that "A
great many of our good people in America support missionaries in India,
maintain hospitals and do other useful work; but as far as I know nobody
has sent out a Dental Surgeon."[11] As a result, some letters detailing missionary activities sought to recruit new dentists: from Meshed, Persia, a physician missionary wrote that "The nearest dentist is Teheran, 600 miles (three
weeks' journey) distant. . . . The essentials for such a dentist are that first, he
or she should be a believing Christian, and, second, a well-trained capable
dentist. Will you not take the matter under consideration?"[12] The Persian
missive was apparently part of a campaign by the Interchurch World Movement to recruit dentists to missionary work: in 1920, *Oral Hygiene* published
a similar press release from the Movement's News Bureau, seeking someone
to introduce "American methods of dentistry" to China.[13]

American Dentistry Abroad

The most pervasive fixation of dental travel writers, whether military or religious, was the state of "American dentistry" abroad. They regarded the esteem
in which American-style dental practice was held, the fees it commanded,
and the ease with which American-trained practitioners could be licensed,
set up their offices, and obtain patients in a foreign country as indicators of
national sagacity (or lack thereof) in the places they visited. They also used

their travels, and their experiences of dental care abroad, to help establish a shared definition of what American dentistry was—principally by describing, with ever more precision, exactly what it was not.

The question of how American dentists themselves would be received in any particular location was not academic. Some published items, intended to help prospective travelers prepare for their stays elsewhere, consisted entirely of summaries of local dental practice laws, with a special emphasis on the possibilities for American practitioners: several prominent American dental journals published periodic updates to their previous compilations of such laws throughout the 1920s. Practice laws favorable to American-trained dentists were remarked upon favorably, though writers disparaged countries in which dental practice was too loosely regulated. "Anybody and everybody, with or without dental education or without any education at all, can set up as a dentist wherever he likes in India," grumbled one dentist. "There is no ordinance nor authority controlling this profession and setting a standard or compelling it to adhere to some professional etiquette, which few [dentists] do."[14] On the other hand, countries whose demanding laws posed barriers to the entry of American practitioners were often openly derided as unnecessarily—and unscientifically—provincial. In 1916, the *Western Dental Journal* informed its readers grumpily that the "chief effect of the new system" of dental licensing in Hong Kong "will be to compel American practitioners to secure British license."[15] Indirectly, these critiques of foreign licensing laws as either too restrictive or too lax helped to forge consensus on the middle range of restraints on practice that might reasonably be applied in the United States.

Dental correspondents often reported on the availability of supplies and competent help abroad (or lack thereof). From Manila, one writer complained of the expense of dental supplies: "There is no dental depot in Manila," he wrote, "but the 'English Drug Store' accommodates (?) the dentists, charging $2.50 to $3.50 for gold and gold solders, $8 per 1/8 oz. for gold pellets, and proportionately high prices for other materials and instruments. It is true that they cost more over there, due to distance and duty charge, bring 20 per cent ad valorem on all dental goods, materials, and instruments."[16] These items were calculated to appeal to budget-minded American dentists, and frequently ran side by side with columns giving advice on how to economize in a domestic dental office. Their authors commented approvingly on countries where dental supplies were reasonably priced, as long as they were also of high quality, or where the locals were willing to fairly remunerate dental work.

Dental travelogues that aimed at recruitment, or at least at getting information to prospective recruits, often concluded with the author's judgment as to the suitability of climate and political life for Americans, and recommendations as to what type of man would be best suited to practice in a particular location. Sometimes the rigor and directness of such analyses undermined recruiting goals: In 1919, for example, James H. Howell reported to the Michigan State Dental Society that "Russia would be a very good place to practice, if, first, you could pass the examination that is required (it must be written in the Russian language); second, if you could speak the language so that you could talk business with your patients; and third, if you could stand to live in the unspeakable conditions in which the country now is."[17]

Good Teeth and Bad Dentistry

Foreign travel frequently provoked dentists' worries about the state of their profession at home, and about the health of Americans' teeth, which they increasingly regarded as reflecting on them. Even the most vicious critics of dental practices abroad had to concur with Weston Price's judgment that the native peoples of many colonized regions had remarkably strong and healthy teeth. "They are in possession of a set of 'ivories' that excite unholy envy in the breast of every white man who sees them," one writer remarked.[18] "A Returned Soldier" wrote in *The Dental Brief* that the Filipino natives had primitive knowledge of dentistry at best, but "the only salvation of the race is that they naturally have good teeth. One may look into the jaws of a hundred natives and find a full set of nice white and sound teeth in each," except for the teeth of women who followed the traditional practice of chewing the betel nut, which stained the teeth red.[19] The condition of Chinese teeth was well known to dental journal readers: the state of the country's dental profession was often commented upon, as in 1903, when *The Dental Brief* reprinted an item from the *Journal of the American Medical Association* stating that "The Chinese have excellent teeth and little use for dentists."[20] Among the isolated natives of Raratonga, too, dental decay was almost unheard of: only 0.3 percent of the natives' teeth had been, as Weston Price put it, "attacked by dental caries."[21]

Unlike Price, however, most dental travel writers focused on the poor state of local dental care, rather than on the excellent health of native people's teeth or the connection between their teeth and their diets. Most American writers agreed that the natives of the places they visited had great teeth in spite of, not because of, the quality of the dental care to which they had access. Native dentistry was defined, in these travelers' minds, by its lack of the very qualities to which these American dentists most aspired—high social and economic status, scientific antisepsis, specificity of remedies and procedures, and efficient business practices—in short, all of the things that made up the evolving vision of professionalism in American dentistry. Dispatches about dentistry abroad, whatever their origins, repeatedly lionized the same American standards of practice, explicitly linking national identity with the quality of dental care, and, eventually, entirely substituting national signifiers for other ways of describing quality dentistry.

Travelers whose work was published in American dental journals complained repeatedly about the poor personal and office hygiene of native dentists. South African dentists used no antiseptic, one writer observed.[22] Native practitioners in India dressed unhygienically, the same correspondent pointed out: during warm months, the native "accommodates himself with a flowing turban, a long coat . . . and a pair of pyjama-like pantaloons. . . . In the winter a thick blanket is added to the costume, this being wrapped across the shoulders according to the method affected by the late Professor Blackie—a modern Greek student with original ideas upon the subject of pronunciation."[23] The resident dentist in Gibraltar used unclean, outdated instruments and seated his white patients in a plush, unhygienic dental chair that "[looked] as though it might have come out of the Ark"; native patients were relegated to a stool in the backyard, in the company of animals.[24] On the other hand, "A Returned Soldier" identified a periphery within a periphery, noting differences between urban and rural dentists in the Philippines that others did not see: "The native dentists in the cities and large towns keep their offices in good order, as a rule, while those in the small towns and barrios are without order."[25]

Criticism of the treatment native dentists doled out to their patients focused heavily on the barbarity of tooth extraction. At home, new developments in bacteriology and materials science contributed to the increasing success of fillings, root canals, and crowns, and to preventing decay from occurring in the first place. As a result, American dentists were coming to see the extraction of diseased teeth as an archaic procedure that could be performed even by the untrained or apprentice-trained, and that was thus beneath the dignity of a truly skilled professional. Extraction represented the failure of dentistry, not its fruition. Accordingly, travel writers stigmatized extraction, and in particular those who seemed to take too much pleasure in performing it. Zulu and Hottentot practitioners, a writer recorded with horror, combined bad hygiene with inappropriate pride in extraction: like "Painless" Parker, they were known to wear the teeth they extracted as jewelry to "adorn their dusky persons."[26] Chinese dentists did the same: "[A]lmost since time immemorial the native operator has drawn attention to his calling by wearing a necklace of teeth to which is attached a cluster of exceptionally formidable molars. If anyone demands proof of the dentist's ability, the operator merely points to his trophies. 'Volumes did not say more.'"[27]

Indiscriminate extraction of teeth offended American dentists as a particular example of native dentists' general lack of commitment to scientific specificity. Western travelers observed with dismay the failure of nonwhite natives to embrace the professional norm of adherence to a specific reductionist school of scientific thought, in which every malady was imagined to have one unique cause and one unique treatment. By comparison, the slipshod diagnostic skills of the natives left Westerners aghast. The Zulu and Hottentot dentists who so proudly wore the results of their labors had frequently extracted the wrong teeth from their patients' mouths, the traveling dentist reported. In such an event, he added, native dentists would then extract the correct teeth for no additional charge. Worst of all, he believed, was that native dentists' lack of commitment to specificity in diagnosis and treatment carried over into their professional self-concepts: in Malta, to his great distress, the native dentists supplemented their income by acting as manicurists, barbers, and chiropodists—the sort of extraprofessional behavior one might have expected of an American dentist a generation before.

Commitment to scientific specificity and to an American-style equality in matters of billing and patient scheduling struck dental travelers as particularly important. One of the most prolific spokesmen for this point of view was British Army dentist George Cecil, who traveled extensively in the British colonies and frequently sent missives tattling on both native and British Army dentists' professional missteps to American dental journals. Cecil shared American dentists' position that high status had to be earned rather than inherited. His resultant support for measures intended to increase the professionalism of dentists everywhere won him particular popularity with American dental journal editors and readers. Over a thirty-year period, Cecil wrote more dental travelogues than any other single author. Many of his articles were reprinted in multiple publications—including some that were republished as many as twenty years after their initial appearances.

Cecil complained bitterly about the languid schedules of native dentists, and of some white dentists in foreign environments. Like many Americans, he was suspicious of "primitive" peoples' alleged disrespect for measured time and for money. On the natives' part, this seemingly blithe disregard for temporality may have been a calculated response to the presence of rude interlopers who made their disrespect for the natives quite plain. During his visit to an Indian dentist in 1891, Cecil was told that his wait for the dentist would be only five minutes, "a period which eventually lengthened into about three-quarters of an hour."[28] On a subsequent visit, Cecil was made to wait for an hour and a half while the dentist took a "siesta."[29] On the dentist's return, Cecil noted acidly, "he seemed considerably surprised that I should have dared to require his services between any hours other than from eight in the morning till midday and from four in the afternoon to seven o'clock in the evening."[30] The reader was left to imagine the interaction that led to the Indian dentist's explanation of his working hours—or, perhaps more likely, not to imagine it. "He is sometimes given to availing himself of holidays in a somewhat unnecessary manner," Cecil wrote of one Anglo-Indian dentist.[31] Patients sometimes traveled great distances to find that their dentist had unexpectedly taken a day off.

Cecil and his American readers shared their perplexity at native dentists' lackadaisical attitude toward the pursuit of profit, and resultant lack of rigor in controlling their own schedules and patients' experiences. When the dentist was present, the patient might be expected to have his treatment enjoyed as a performance by spectators: Zulus and Hottentots extracted teeth from their countrymen "in the presence of all the inhabitants for miles around."[32] Patients in many locales could expect to be dealt with in order of their social prominence—a fact which particularly irked Cecil. "Any unfortunate native patients who happen to be on the premises at the time are unceremoniously bundled out into the street or told to wait until 'His Greatness' has been attended to," he complained.[33] Cecil regarded attempts by dentists to treat white patients preferentially with similar scorn, for they revealed the same unprofessional tendency to discriminate between patients on the basis of social power.

Cecil also expected patients to observe the modern American norms of doctor-patient interaction, and found native patients—wherever he went—deficient in this skill. In South Africa, Cecil observed that black Africans with toothaches often combined their visits to the dentist with travels related to trade. The Africans, he reported, felt free to "wriggle" off the dental stool in the middle of treatment to transact their business with the white man on whose veranda the itinerant dentist had set up shop.[34] What non-white natives failed to complain about was just as significant a sign to Cecil: South African patients, he imagined, greeted with excitement infection and pain so excruciating that it interfered with alimentation. The "[Kaffir] hails with delight any opportunity of imbibing the cheap and poisonous whiskey which is sold by the missionary element."[35] Cecil's analysis found purchase with American dentists who regarded people of African ancestry as insensate to pain (or, alternatively—and incoherently—as persons who were constantly looking for an opportunity to drug themselves into insensibility).[36] He was equally disquieted by natives' casualness in paying for dental services. Rich Indians, he observed, "are excellent customers to the dentist, [but] they are not what may be described as 'good pay.' In point of fact they are the most dishonest rascals conceivable. To lie and cheat appears to be part of their religion, and as far as carrying out the observance in question is concerned they may be said to be singularly pious."[37] The "Rajah," Cecil commented, would promise payment and fail to deliver, and the Indian bureaucracy— both white and native—was so corrupt that it was impossible to use the law to compel the wayward patient to pay. The patient might even pretend that he had died in order to duck his bill, Cecil observed, and "one native being so very like another that it is often a matter of difficulty to tell them apart," the dentist would not be able to provide proof to the contrary.[38] Cecil therefore grudgingly approved of demanding cash in advance of services rendered, a practice widely regarded as the mainstay of charlatans in the United States, and which Cecil might have received as evidence of the brutalizing influence of the Indian environment had it not involved the securing of payment. Cecil did note that the officers of native and British regiments were not much more reliable debtors than non-military patients. Anglo-Indian officers' wives, he said, were in the habit of offering sex in lieu of payment for dental services, so that they might be able to use the allowances their husbands gave them for "the purchase of finery" instead of dental treatment.[39] How he had come upon this information was also left unsaid.

Cecil's and other travelers' observations on the widespread failure to observe American professional norms indicted the British as well as the colonized natives themselves. These writers' excursions into colonized territories gave American dentists, as both writers and readers, the opportunity to compare their practices not only with those of the natives but with those of the British colonizers of those locales, staking out an imagined professional territory distant from either place. The British suffered in the comparison. American dentist Landis Wirt, reporting from Bangalore, observed that among the British, dentists' social status was not appreciably better than that of workingmen. "It is not generally admitted that British gentlemen's sons enter the dental profession as it would mean loss of cast [sic]. Therefore the British profession depends for its recruits mostly on the inferior classes. But in America, dentistry is held an honorable calling and the sons of many of our best citizens enter it, thus bringing to it a high type of intellect."[40] In 1911, the high social status of dentistry in the United States was by no means uniform; Wirt's jingoism was as much an attempt to influence reality as to reflect it. Then, too, he was participating in the popular American denigration of British imperialism on the grounds of its alleged obsession with status and class. American imperialism, such critics thought, was more rational, and more just.

George Cecil echoed Wirt's criticisms of British dentistry: the British Army, he complained in 1913, accepted only recruits whose jaws were in perfect condition, and then dedicated itself to their destruction. Soldiers, required to keep their equipment and surroundings spotless, were never asked to clean their teeth, and the barracks in which they lived were wet, cold, and ill-ventilated, setting the stage for health disaster. Rough, unpalatable food magnified these troubles. Dental care was unavailable: "The average army doctor has only one method of treating toothache. It is that of extraction."[41] Though Cecil claimed to be trying to change this state of affairs on his own (in part, at least, through shining the purifying light of public attention upon it), he asserted that the vanity and social climbing of Royal Army Medical Corps doctors made real change unlikely. "For, what time remains over from taking care of his uniform, admiring his sword, brushing his moustache, cultivating a military bearing and the acquaintance of his social superiors, is not devoted by the medical man in question to studying his profession."[42] Local English doctors in India, in Cecil's evaluation, had even more laughable skills than their native dental professional counterparts: "The last-named," he noted with respect to these Englishmen, "in his general knowledge of dentistry, is rather less than primitive. An intelligent butcher would do almost as well."[43]

British and native dentists' pretenses to dental skill did reveal one nugget of good judgment for which Cecil, like other dental travel writers, praised them: everywhere, it seemed, dentists esteemed American dental practice. Cecil observed that the native Indian population, and especially the Anglo-Indian population, was attracted (sometimes deceptively) by the promise of American dental technology. "American dentistry is much in favor at the moment, the Anglo-Indian community becoming a convert to its advantages every day."[44] And: "A considerable number of dentists practicing in India put on their plates the title 'American Dentist,' thus hoping to catch those clients who are likely to be attracted thereby. As a matter of fact their work does not resemble that of America's leading dental exponents."[45] By the nineteen-teens, American dentistry was held in such high esteem that one Egyptian dental practitioner could write that "Everyone knows that in Europe American dentistry stands for what is best and what is worst. The popularity and success of the first American dentists there brought out a crop of fake American dentists who had never even seen the States." He went further in his negative assessment of British dentists' abilities: "I have had under my care English, Scotch, and Irish soldiers and officers, Australians, New Zealanders, and Canadians too, and I could easily tell at a glance—just a superficial survey of the mouth— whether the patient hailed from the British colonies or the British Isles. The latter presented as a rule the most appalling conditions. . . . this condition is not to be blamed on the 'high-class American dentistry,' but on American dentistry as practiced in England."[46] Even in backward China, the same held true: "Despite their boasts, the Chinese have not been slow in recognizing the superiority of American dentistry."[47]

Explicit references to the superiority of American dental practice, as judged either by the peoples on whom dental travel writers reported or by the travelers themselves, constituted a genre within a genre. American dental travel writers described the history of professional dentistry (which one writer identified as beginning with the 1839 establishment of the Baltimore College of Dental Surgery) as a uniquely American story: "The efficient practice of dentistry, then as now," wrote N. S. Jenkins in 1917, "required a high standard of technical skill and resourcefulness. Owing to physical and social conditions, Americans have always shown a special aptitude and inventiveness in the mechanic arts, and these hereditary qualities gave them for a considerable time a superiority in the practice of dentistry."[48] Jenkins, drawing on his own fifty-year residence in Europe, explained that American dentists who practiced in Europe were at an advantage because of their progress through the true meritocracy of the United States. "Coming from a country where caste was unknown," he wrote, "[their] social positions and influence [were] entirely dependent upon [their] breeding and character." Surveying the range of travel undertaken and reported on by Americans, he concluded that, despite the passage of immigration laws restricting the movement of Europeans into the United States, the cross-fertilization of the profession in

Europe by Americans and "the conditions which have made American dentistry such a power for good in the world will endure."[49]

Later writers confirmed the accuracy of his prediction, as they described foreign dentists' and governments' promotion of American-style dentistry. In 1923, the government-sponsored *Military Dental Journal* reported that the recent Japan earthquake had decimated a burgeoning American-style dental program: "It was only a little over a year ago that Prof. Chiwaki—who contributed nearly all of his personal fortune and a lifetime of energy toward the establishment, along American lines, of the Tokyo Dental College—came to this country in quest of fresh educational ideas." the article mourned. "Japan, Chiwaki says, owes many things to America, dentistry being one of them. Japanese dentistry is an outgrowth of our own."[50] In 1920, E. C. Kirk of Philadelphia reported to the Connecticut Dental Hygiene Association that the British had rebounded from the Great War and had dedicated a large amount of public money to the establishment of oral hygiene programs. "This old British world, which we have at times regarded as a little bit stodgy and slower than ourselves, has wakened up, and is doing great things," he said. Then he interposed, reaffirming the supremacy of American leadership in dentistry: "America is after all the source, the origin, of many of the biggest things in dentistry."[51]

Travel writers felt it a matter of great importance that the United States be recognized for its peculiar dental prowess. They also did the important work of reminding American dentists to adhere to the new professional practices that were slowly but certainly making American dentistry so successful— and so different from dentistry as it was practiced everywhere else. Their penchant for portraying themselves as the arbiters of who or what could be denominated "American" helped to cement the link between American national identity and the pursuit of ever-improved, ever-complex dental interventions. Eventually, this connection helped to shape dentists' responses to the prospects of incorporating particular new territories and peoples into the United States, and to influence popular ideas about what ideas and attitudes about dentistry and teeth could be described as American.

The Philippines

The Philippines, colonized by the United States after the Spanish-American War, were an important destination for dental travelers. Most Philippine dental travelers were connected to the United States military or to the civil government established in the Philippines, and headed by US elites including William Howard Taft, after the close of the war. The density of the US military presence in the Philippines was due partly to the Filipinos' continuing resistance to US occupation—between 1899 and 1902, Filipinos fought a fierce guerrilla war against American forces, during which 220,000 Filipinos and 4,500 Americans were killed.[52] The intensity of Filipino resistance, and the strategic importance of the Philippines to the United States, resulted in a continual infusion of American troops—and dentists who treated them—into the islands. There, the identification of dentistry with Americanism would usually work to support arguments against annexation, which were prevalent throughout popular commentary on the Philippines at the time.

Dentist writers immediately complained of the degraded state of dental practice in the Philippines. "A Returned Soldier" noted in 1902 that native dentists in the Philippine countryside were part-time practitioners, "who work in the fields, and practise their profession only when called upon to do so."[53] Such dental workers, "many wearing the breech-cloth," used crude instruments: "Returned Solider" included a full page of sketched examples, including an indicting example of the natives' "advertising ideas," a large tooth made from wood and designed to clatter against the dentist's signboard "to attract the attention of persons passing by."[54] As from so many other locales, this dental traveler reported that despite the conditions of native dental practice, the Filipinos had beautiful and healthy teeth, only occasionally marred by the chewing of betel nuts or the use of tobacco.

Dental travelers to the Philippines were soon to initiate a more colorful and—from the standpoint of American imperialists—more ominous series of reports. Like the Americans and Filipino collaborationist governors themselves, these writers discovered that among the knottiest problems in the colonization of the islands was the lack of cooperation of the "savage" and "barbaric" tribes living in parts of the Philippines.[55] The guerrilla warfare that plagued the cause of American imperialism was carried out in part by these tribespeople, who had never been pacified by Spanish colonial rule and resisted vigorously the prospect of pacification by Americans. Dental travel writers pointed to the aesthetic appearance of the natives' teeth, and their attitudes toward American-style dentistry, as evidence of their lack of assimilability to American culture and ways of self-government. The tribesmen's teeth would provide, alternately, evidence of the need for American "help" to the Filipino "little brown brother," and proof that the US excursion in the Philippines was ultimately futile.

In 1904, "A Regular" informed readers of *The Dental Review* that the "Mohammedan" chiefs of Mindanao, "heretofore invincible" headhunters, "endeavor[ed] to make [their] features as disgusting and as frightful as possible, for the purpose of designating [their] ideas and for scaring and confusing [their] foe[s] when the two meet in combat. The result is that you can meet with some really frightful looking mouths."[56] "Regular" also included sketches of teeth that had been filed to points, set with pearls, dyed black, bored through and linked together with gold wire rings, or yanked from an enemy's severed head and worn as jewelry (in this instance, a molar mounted in a ring setting with its roots protruding perpendicularly from the wearer's finger).

A final section of the text, optimistically titled "Americans Changing These Ideas," reported that American soldiers "desire that this head hunting idea be stopped," and had arrested some "fanatics." The concluding paragraph also made vague and brief references to "better order" and the establishment of "trails to lake regions" to facilitate the extraction of natural resources: there was no comment on American interest in (or success at) stopping tooth decoration or mutilation practices.[57]

The community of American dentists in the Philippines was a close-knit one, and their familiarity with one another's reports to American dental journals was high. In 1905, Manila dentist Louis Ottofy, an American who practiced for twenty-three years in the Philippines and Japan, informed readers of *The Dental Cosmos* that he had been "unable to confirm" the reports of "A Returned Soldier" and "A Regular" about the state of dentistry among the native Filipinos and tribes. Ottofy emphasized instead the marginal success of attempts to establish Western-style dental services in the Philippines. These attempts, he felt, were impeded by warfare, linguistic and educational barriers, and natural disaster—not surprisingly, the same forces that hampered US imperial aspirations in the region more generally. His cautious expression of hopes for the future reflected the tenuousness of the American government's hold on the situation in the Philippines. After a litany of the disasters that had befallen the islands, he zeroed in on the effects of these disasters on crops, which had "often [been] totally destroyed by a plague of locusts, and by various insects attacking the coffee plant and other vegetation. Happily, the Islands are now practically free from these scourges, and very little is now feared, except possibly from the locusts. It is not too optimistic to predict that the Islands are now entering on an era of prosperity."[58]

Ottofy feared that the prosperity for which he hoped (barring a return of the locusts) might be delayed or prevented by the lack of dental services in

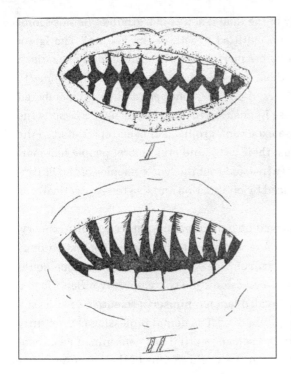

Figure 4 Teeth of Philippine Moro headhunters, as portrayed by "A Regular" in 1904. *Dental Review* 18 (April 15, 1904): 319.

the Philippines. In fact, he took the comparatively radical step of suggesting that, until a dental school could be established, "native young men" could be trained "toward the giving of relief in remote sections of the country, the introduction of simple fillings, and substitution of the teeth when lost."[59] In the context of American dentists' home-front anxieties about gaining and maintaining professional status, and particularly as part of a genre of literature that repeatedly emphasized the importance of establishing American-style dental practice regulations abroad, Ottofy's willingness to entertain the idea of training Filipino natives in some facets of dentistry was unusual and significant. Dentists like Ottofy conceived of American credibility and success in its Pacific colonies as resting in part on the ability to disseminate American dentistry, regardless of the cost to the image of American dentistry as being exemplified by thorough education and training. Sometimes the imperatives of colonialism won out over the imperatives of professionalization.

Ottofy himself seemed particularly invested in the notion that adherence to American standards of dental appearance would be an important index of the assimilability of the Filipinos to an American way of life. Three years later, he published a massive study of the dental status of a group of Bontoc Igorot tribespeople of northern Luzon, entitled "Teeth of the Igorots." The Igorot were already familiar, not only to American dentists but to many American laypeople. Several groups of them had been brought to the United States to serve as exhibits in World's Fairs, the most prominent and best-remembered of them the Louisiana Purchase Exposition in St. Louis in 1904.[60] Despite the fact that the members of these excursion groups had been repatriated to the Philippines (sometimes against their will), and other Igorot people had married Christian Filipinos, Ottofy insisted that the Igorot peoples of the Philippines "ha[ve] not been influenced by civilization and live today practically as [they] did in ages gone by."[61]

Ottofy was profoundly moved by contemporary anthropological theory. He described his travels into the territory inhabited by the Bontoc Igorot as a reversed recapitulation of the history of civilization, in which one could observe an almost evolutionary regression from contemporary urban life to a more primitive past lifestyle. He also fancied himself a scientist, or at least a competent critic of science, arguing that "The dental profession cannot fully justify its claim that dentistry is a science until it has determined what people, if any, possess the best teeth in the world."[62] One of the purposes of his article was to cement the scientific credentials of the dental profession: the most persistent theme of his report was that, despite difficulty in examining Igorot children, he had become certain that "the Igorot has not only the best teeth in the world, but far better ones than had been supposed to exist among any people at the present time."[63]

Ottofy's most important role was as an ambassador between the Igorot peoples and his own American readers, and he performed this function avidly. He complained that other travel writers had misrepresented the Philippines and their inhabitants: "much that is erroneous and absolutely false is spread broadcast by ignorant men, who visit the islands, live at Manila, seldom go anywhere else, and, when they do, have not the ability or intelligence to carefully observe what they see."[64] He shared the belief that the respectful observance of American norms of dental aesthetics was an important index of civilization (or at least of the potential for it). He disagreed with other informants about the state of such observance in the Philippines. First among his targets for debunking was the widely circulated claim that the "Igorot and Negrito tribes of northwestern Luzon take special delight in filing their teeth to a point."[65] Ottofy presented a series of objections to this claim: "In the first place, there are no Negritos in northwestern Luzon, secondly, Igorots do not mar their teeth in any manner."[66] Though he did concede that the Negritos had been known to chip away (not file) sections of their teeth, he insisted that the Igorots had never engaged in this, or any other, tooth-altering practice.

Ottofy believed that the Igorot people, though barbarian, had in common with Americans their insistence on keeping their natural (and, in the case of the Igorot, very healthy) teeth intact. The next section of his report on the "Teeth of the Igorots" included a lengthy and seemingly out-of-place paean to the geographic formations of the Philippines, which, he argued, were remarkably similar to those in the United States. "Much of it seemed to me like what I have seen in the Alleghenies and the Cascades, and then again rugged like the Rockies and the Sierra Nevadas, with spots of beauty like those in the Blue Mountain range."[67] Taken together, these twin examples of forced comparison between the Philippines and the United States illuminate the project of Ottofy's report: he was interested not only in documenting the dental status of the Igorot, but also in contributing to a popular construction of the Philippines as a place fundamentally similar to the United States. Many of the military and civil governors of the Philippines had been "Indian fighters" before being deployed abroad, and much of the discourse around the Pacific colonies of the United States figured those colonies as representing trans-Pacific extensions of Manifest Destiny. In the Philippines as in North America, this narrative suggested, Americans had subdued a diverse and beautiful landscape, and had pacified noble yet barbaric peoples. Ottofy's description of the teeth of the Igorot was of a piece with this discourse, and suggests that for him, embrace of Americans' high standards of dental appearance was an important index of this pacification, or susceptibility to it.[68]

Despite Ottofy's claims, reports of dental depravity in the Philippines—and, particularly, of dental decoration and mutilation in Luzon—persisted.[69] Other writers insisted that the peoples of the Philippines were beyond the reaches of missionary attempts to instill in them a healthy respect for the Protestant work ethic. S. D. Boak snidely remarked that "'Our little brown brothers' have the art of living without work well brought down to a science."[70] Where the "little brown brother" trope included the possibility that Filipinos, on maturing to "adulthood," could be safely brought into the family of the United States, Boak held out little hope for that eventuality. After telling a recalcitrant Filipino that "we Caucasians look upon work as the highest and holiest thing there is, and the greatest purifier that the world has known," Boak was startled to be asked why, if Americans so prized work, "the workers are the most despised and most miserable, and invariably receive their share of worldly wealth and goods from the small end of the horn? . . . If manual labor, or work. . . . is so purifying and exalting, why is it that the one ambition of the Caucasian is to acquire enough wealth so as he can live without laboring?"[71] Boak reported that "[this] philosophy took [his] breath." Boak's attention—and his readers'—was distracted from this question and its critique of the American socioeconomic system by the sense of righteous vindication he experienced when the questioner proceeded to catch and eat a locust that had just flown by, "calmly [remarking], 'The Lord always provides.'"[72] Such reports, touching as they did on Americans' most diligently observed taboos (including the taboo against ingesting the flesh of certain animals; many writers titillated their readers by announcing the Igorots' alleged predilection for eating dog) highlighted the radically unassimilable culture of the natives of the Philippines.

Later writers did file cautiously optimistic reports about the accommodations being struck between American dental practices and those of Philippine natives. The allegedly fierce Islamic Moro tribesmen, for example, had by 1922 "relax[ed] somewhat in some of their radical practices," and had "added the tooth brush and a tube of paste to their list of toilet articles."[73] At least for a time, relations between the Americans and the Moros (some of whom served in the American-led military of the Philippines) did soften. Christian Filipinos settled in Moro lands, and the presence of Americans apparently served to repress conflicts between the two groups. But the Americans' insistence on segregating the Christians and the Moros led to disaster after the establishment of the Philippine Commonwealth in 1935. After years of separation, Moros thought of themselves as fundamentally different from Christian Filipinos and objected to being ruled by them.[74]

American dental travel writers in the Philippines considered both the dental health and the dental practices of Filipinos to be useful indices of the success, or likelihood of success, of US imperialism in the Pacific. They peppered their descriptions of the natives' teeth with observations on the cultural, dietary, and labor practices of the Philippines because they thought of these things as being fundamentally related to one another. A long-running tension between those who thought of US imperialism as the natural outgrowth of Manifest Destiny and those who considered the Filipino peoples themselves immovable obstacles to American aspirations in the Pacific, and racially unassimilable, played itself out in the way that American dental travelers wrote about the islands and their inhabitants. The writing of most dentists who spent time in the Philippines bore the markings of a profound sense of despair about the possibility that the Philippines could become American. Racially, culturally, geographically, and dentally, the people of the Philippines were simply not similar enough to the people of the United States. These writings, by defining what was not, and could never be, American, helped to define what was American in the process. Though US domination of the Philippines continued, objections like the ones raised by these travel writers would play a part in scuttling the annexation of the Philippines to the United States.

Hawai'i

Like the Philippines, the islands of Hawai'i were the focus of much American interest in the early decades of the twentieth century. The islands had been colonized in the late 1800s by American sugar companies and, after the 1898 US-sponsored overthrow of the Hawai'ian monarch Queen Lili'uokalani in 1900, by the US government itself.[75] One of the earliest American dentists to travel to colonial Hawai'i reported extensively in 1901 about the perils of the journey (chiefly seasickness) and about the beautiful natural features of the islands he visited. In keeping with the American tradition of minimizing the visibility and significance of the locals who had inhabited areas that would become American states, Sacramento dentist F. H. Metcalf commented only that "The people are most hospitable and vie with each other in giving the tourist a good time."[76] It may have been that Metcalf was referring to white inhabitants of Hawai'i rather than to native Hawai'ians themselves, however, for his next sentence read: "I found my professional brethren progressive, up to date, and a bunch of good fellows." Metcalf also minimized the subject of the professional meeting he attended in Hawai'i, describing it only as "alive with interest and good fellowship, and a programme of which will be sent to you by the secretary."[77] His report was part of the subgenre of dental travel writing that sought to promote class-appropriate vacations for American dentists, but it was also among a steady stream of dental travel writing specifically concerned with Hawai'i. Unlike Metcalf's, however, almost all of the later reports from Hawai'i by dentists contained much more extensive meditations on the differences between Hawai'i and the United States, and speculation about whether and how those differences could be bridged.

The racial similarities and differences between Hawai'i and the United States were foremost among the concerns of dentists who traveled and practiced in the islands. In fact, some speculated that the multi- but not interracial character of Hawai'ian society made it an ideal laboratory for the testing

of contemporary dental and social theories. Three American dentists living in Hawai'i introduced a five-part series of articles on dental disease in
the islands with the proviso that "It seems to us that the most promising
approach to problems concerning dentition is through comparative studies
of racial groups living under comparable hygienic conditions. Hawai'i offers
a rare opportunity for study of this kind. . . . Many races are residents on the
islands and live together in close proximity, yet to a large extent maintain
their racial customs and food habits. . . . The social service work of the territory is highly organized and through the various centers entrée can be had
to every village and to practically every home."[78] Their words gestured to the
importance of race to contemporary Americans, as well as to the writers' optimism that the Hawai'ian experiment of careful racial mingling of persons of
Native Hawai'ian, Japanese, Chinese, Filipino, and European descent might
hold valuable lessons for the similar American experiment underway on the
mainland, particularly in the American West. Most importantly, the articles
referenced the writers' solidarity with, and intent to make use of, the "social
service work of the territory," including a centralized system of primary and
secondary education, all aimed at uplifting and improving the lives of native
Hawai'ians, willingly or no.

This commingling of Americanization campaigns and professional
American dentistry would continue on the Hawai'ian islands throughout
the first half of the twentieth century. In Honolulu, the Palama settlement
included a well-funded and much remarked-upon dental clinic, and other
Americanization regimens incorporated dental care as a prominent part of
their programs. Dental travelers to Hawai'i often pointed to the Palama (or
"Paloma") settlement's dental clinic, which ran from 1914 until 1921 when
it was replaced by the Honolulu Dental Infirmary for Children, as a model
for future clinic projects. In 1930, supervising dental hygienist Helen Baukin
reported on the Kapaa school dental program at Kauai, listing among the
school staff not only teachers and principals, but a "nutrition worker," dentist
and dental hygienist, government physician, deputy sheriff, probation officer,
sanitation officer, and juvenile court judge. (Baukin offered no comment as to
why the school required such a strong police presence; mainland schools of
comparable size did not typically host such an array of law enforcement personnel.) Her article, published in the *Journal of the American Dental Association*, highlighted the establishment of a daily "toothbrush drill" (illustrated
by a photograph in the article) as among the most important innovations of
the curriculum. In the photo, native Hawai'ian students stood in uneven lines

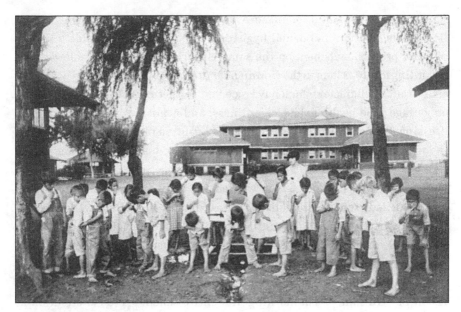

Figure 5 Children on the front lawn of the Kapaa School participate in a "toothbrush drill," 1930. *Journal of the American Dental Association* 17 (February 1930): 359. Copyright © 1930 American Dental Association. All rights reserved. Reprinted by permission.

on the front lawn of their school building, leaning gamely into all the various attitudes of toothbrushing.

The toothbrush "drill" was not the only Kapaa School manifestation of coercive American colonialism in Hawai'i. The school lunch program, described in the lunchroom bulletin as "Army Chow," also bore explicit hallmarks of military posturing. The lunchroom was crowded, one issue of the bulletin acknowledged, but the situation called for everyone's patience and obedience: "Order Best," read the headline on the item. The principal had banned the use of white rice in the school kitchen, preferring the more nutritious brown rice though "the storekeepers could not understand how anyone could possibly prefer the brown rice to the clean white kernels, nor did the parents see the wiseness of the change."[79] Students were provided with hot lunches at the school, the better to "teach them the use of table utensils as well as proper table manners."[80] The lunchroom flyer also extolled the virtues of the Vocational Homemaking Class, which had recently graduated seven young women. "We hope them further success in life. They know how to cook and sew—that's a great deal."[81]

In their attempts to inculcate American values through Hawai'i's public schools, dentists and dental hygienists took their places beside a variety of other professionals bent on the same end. Hawai'i's white teachers were, according to a 1923 item in the *Hawaii Educational Review*, expected to emphasize "traits of character which have received least attention at home. They can encourage good health habits, cleanliness, and neatness, and modest, simple dressing; they can instill a regard for civic beauty, a respect for human values in law and order and property rights, and they can hold up high standards of living."[82] Patriotic rituals figured heavily into these school-based Americanization campaigns: teachers who worked in Hawai'ian schools in the 1920s and 1930s led "school assemblies emphasizing loyalty, saluting the flag and singing patriotic songs."[83] As in the mainland school hygiene programs, in Hawai'i the principles of the dental hygiene and health programs made natural counterparts to the civic virtues schools sought to inculcate in their students. "Loyalty to his fellowmen as well as to his country, is greatly stressed," Helen Baukin said, "Each morning, the entire school stands at attention as the Stars and Stripes are raised, and with unfaltering voices, these children of numerous races pledge allegiance to Old Glory. For the outsider, whose privilege it is to be present at the Flag raising exercises, the heart beats faster to hear the many children of many ages and races slowly and emphatically pledge." Baukin ended her report with the text of the Pledge of Allegiance.[84] Kapaa School students were being introduced to American nationalism and American dentistry with the same educational program: loyalty to "his country" [the United States] was explicitly linked for the Kapaa student with the use of the toothbrush.

As the inauguration of Hawai'ian statehood approached, dental travel writers grew even more optimistic about the prospects for the seamless incorporation of the territory into the fabric of the American nation. H. Dorothy Dudley wrote to Michigan dentists in 1936 that "Dental practice is no different in Hawaii from dental practice in Michigan. Caries, malocclusions and periodonticlasia are universal, as recent surveys in all parts of the world have established. In civilized communities the statistics for the different age-groups vary very little. And Hawaii is civilized. (I have seen grass skirts *only* in shop windows for tourists, and it is said they are made in Grand Rapids.)"[85] Dudley's use of the term "civilized" was clarified by her description of the changes wrought on traditional Hawai'ian eating practices by dental public health nurses: "Some portion of the high rice diet eaten by most Oriental families has been replaced by other foods which contain more of the food elements necessary for building and maintaining good teeth. The Classical Public Health teaching of: More milk, more fruit, more vegetables and whole grain bread has had a demonstrable effect."[86] Her emphasis on the modification of Hawai'ian eating practices to a more Western model suggests that she meant not that Hawai'i was, inherently, a civilized place, but that it *had been civilized* (by American intervention). Her comparison of dentistry in Hawai'i to dentistry in Michigan was calculated not only to appeal to the readers of the Michigan state dental journal, but, by its claim that Hawai'i was no different from an existing American state, to advance the case for Hawai'ian statehood.

A 1938 item in the merged *Journal of the American Dental Association/Dental Cosmos* presented evidence of a fully operational school dental hygiene program being implemented in Hawai'ian schools on the model of the best of civilized "American" dentistry. Dental hygienists were being trained "after the Bridgeport, Conn. Plan," receiving two years of essential "basic cultural and scientific background" followed by two years of dental hygiene education and a final year of public health training. The hygienists had been properly authorized by Hawai'ian law to practice in the territory's public schools, and twenty-five were working in those schools at the time of the article. Hygienists used modern, portable equipment, and kept "definite records of each child." An award program had been developed to recognize school classes with the fastest achievement of "100 percent dental correction."[87] These formalities of law and professional practice were of central importance to American dentists, and the American Dental Association's report that they were being observed in Hawai'i signaled the organization's belief that the imposition of a rational, scientific, American model of dental practice—and political life—was not only possible, but well underway, which boded well for the cause of statehood.

Interest in the success of Americanization in Hawai'i persisted until well beyond Hawai'i's admission to the union in 1959. In 1964, for example, an article in *Dental Students' Magazine* marked the transition visually, showcasing photographs of the modern Ala Moana building, "a popular location for dental offices," as well as of a Honolulu dentist's modern "operatory," and a tastefully decorated Honolulu reception room where "live bamboo and orchids accentuate the Polynesian décor." Hawai'ian dentists, James Voigt wrote, were rigorously trained and tested, and later enrolled responsibly in their state and county dental associations, which "[enjoyed] a 98 per cent participation." There was, he wrote, "no dental advertising in the state." Such advertising would have been superfluous, Voigt suggested: "Hawai'i's present dental needs," he assured student readers, "are adequately met with the modern techniques that are practiced in the Islands' many private offices and dental clinics." In physical plant as in business and professional practice, Hawai'ians had exceeded the threshold of Americanness.[88]

The writings generated by American dental travelers to Hawai'i formed a narrative of cautious optimism leading to a joyful intertwining of American and Hawai'ian identities and interests. Of course, the process of colonization in Hawai'i was far more complicated—and more contested—than articles written from the *haole* (white) point of view tend to suggest. But these items illustrate how American dentists thought of their roles in the propagation of American values and American culture in this American territory. These writers used the indices of American dentistry—measures of professionalization like recordkeeping and licensure, and standards of bourgeois American taste as applied to office décor and participation in public political ritual—to gauge the potential and actual success of Hawai'ians in living up to the American standards set by their colonizers. Given the involvement of other professionals, like teachers, in such enterprises, dentists' interest in encouraging and charting Americanization should not be surprising. It illustrates with specificity the function of American dental travel writing: such texts worked to facilitate the symmetry of American identity with a positive vision of dental practice and patienthood.

It was hard for dentists to explain, to themselves or to anyone else, why a country with the best, most scientifically advanced dental profession in the world remained populated by people with such terrible teeth. Americans' continued bad dental health severely tested claims of their genetic, cultural, and political superiority to other nationalities, and seriously disrupted the idea that "American" always meant something positive. In the middle of the twentieth century, it also caused Americans to press for dental care that was more accessible and affordable, heightening the national clamor for the socialization of health care costs and posing a threat to the financial success and professional autonomy dentists had so recently won.

Chapter 4

"This National Stupidity"

American Dental Economics in the 1930s and 1940s

"Gentlemen," one Boston dentist admonished his colleagues at a professional conference in 1949, "I believe that the seductive delusion and blandishments of a 'heaven on earth' philosophy is intriguing and undermining the traditional sane thinking of America." The Truman administration's postwar plan for national health insurance, he thought, was leading Americans down a primrose path to socialism. "Only by aggressively applying your superior talents and the knowledge acquired through your education in the fight against this national stupidity," he counseled, "can you settle your balance with your community, your state and your nation."[1]

By the middle of the twentieth century, American dentists generally shared their Boston colleague's sense of the profession as a justifiably elite occupation and of its practitioners as men of special intelligence and perspicacity. Dentists took pride in the technical achievements of the discipline, and in their voluntary contributions to the health of American children through school hygiene programs and recommendations about diet. In raising the status of the profession, they had also increased their ability to command payment. Dentists' incomes rose accordingly. When dental care was provided to a patient for free, the dentist involved had either been paid from public coffers or made a voluntary decision to be charitable. As the Boston dentist warned, however, dentists faced mounting anger from fellow citizens who were angered by their lack of access to dental services during the Depression, and by the inadequate number and distribution of dentists during the boom in demand for services caused by World War II.

State and federal legislators reacted to these failures of the market by pro-
posing plans of health and dental insurance that caused dentists to fear for
their professional autonomy. Together with the example of physicians who
successfully organized against such programs, this fear helped to persuade
most dentists that maintaining the cherished system of private payment
against the "national stupidity" of dental insurance was not only possible,
but essential. As a result, federal and state efforts to provide a safety net of
guaranteed health and dental benefits to children, the elderly, and the poor
met with vehement opposition from the dentists of the ADA.

Charity Care

Both physicians and dentists had long tried to limit the opportunities for
Americans to receive health care outside of the private-payer system. Physicians were particularly successful in opposing programs for free care to the
indigent. Though poor health among the impoverished, particularly among
women and children, inspired the creation of the federal Children's Bureau
in 1910 and the 1921 passage of the Sheppard-Towner Act which provided
for health screenings and education oriented towards maternal and child
health, the AMA's lobbying prevented either program from including funding for direct medical care. In the nineteen-teens, the American Association
for Labor Legislation aggressively promoted plans of income protection for
industrial workers sidelined by illness or injury, pointing to the notorious
bad health of applicants for military service as a way to justify such plans as a
national interest. Partly in order to avoid the AMA's opposition to these plans,
however, the AALL did not contemplate the payment of physician bills.[2] Physicians frequently staffed free or low-cost dispensary clinics, either on a vol-
unteer basis or for pay; but they insisted that dispensary services be made
available only to the very poorest Americans, reasoning that those who could
afford to pay for medical care ought to be made to do so.

　　Early twentieth-century dentists faced a professional climate somewhat
more hostile than the one physicians confronted. Unlike physicians, they
had not yet succeeded in consolidating in the mind of the public the image of
their profession as the high-status provider of an invaluable health service.
The broad popular following of "Painless" Parker, who derided the ADA as
a trust designed to create a monopoly market for American dentists, threatened dentists' hopes to create a climate of exclusivity around the profession,
and dentists were willing to provide a certain amount of free care to keep
anti-monopolists off their backs. School dental hygiene programs were an

important part of this effort, but the limitation of their services to children left a large gap in available care for adults.

Like physicians, many dentists attempted to address the shortfall in care available to adults by contributing their time, sometimes without pay, to free or low-cost public dispensaries. Even the most fervent proponents of dentists' participation in such arrangements agreed that free care should be available only to the very poorest patients. In 1913, for example, Boston dentist Frederick Keyes told the members of the Guild of St. Apollonia that physicians had erred in making dispensary care too freely available, and that dentists ought to guard their own charitable contributions of time more closely. "The free dental dispensary is just as essential for the health of the public as the free medical dispensary," he wrote. "Similarly, the work should be done gratis. But its scope should be limited as far as possible to the treatment of the worthy poor."[3] Others shared Keyes's conviction that free care ought to be focused on those whose poverty was through no fault of their own, "so as not to interfere with the legitimate rights of private practitioners or to compromise those people so bitterly opposed to any form of socialistic measures," and argued that the dentists providing it ought to be paid consultants rather than volunteers.[4] This, they felt, would help to avoid "any disorderly arrangement of operations as is wont to occur when volunteers give their time spasmodically and work in a haphazard manner," and to promote the competitive selection of candidates for dispensary employment, which would help to improve the state of dentistry overall.[5]

Industrial Dental Hygiene Programs

Because dentists generally preferred opportunities to work for pay, they usually avoided low- or unpaid dispensary work, focusing their energies on more remunerative programs. Among the most vaunted were industrial hygiene programs providing dental service to American workers. In the early decades of the twentieth century, as the American industrial economy exploded, manufacturing employers hoped to prevent the disruptions of production that ensued when employees suffering dental pain failed to appear for work, or worked less efficiently than they might have had they been healthy. Slowdowns like these posed particular problems for American employers during years in which preparation for and prosecution of war meant that American factories were otherwise operating at full capacity. To remediate this problem, dentists promoted campaigns of dental inspection and treatment sponsored by employers for workers. Thaddeus P. Hyatt, the dental director of Metropolitan Life Insurance Company, argued that health problems of all sorts, and resultant time away from work, were significantly decreased by such programs. "There is no question but what industrial dental clinics will prove of great value to the country," he wrote, "The only question that it is necessary to firmly establish is the fact that it is good business for large companies to establish these dental clinics."[6] In Cleveland, Weston Price produced a copiously illustrated talk directed at company managers, intended to persuade them of the necessity of providing dental care in their facilities and featuring before-and-after photographs of a young man crippled by dental disease and then cured through a dentist's intervention. "Can we say of this generation that management was not responsible because they did not know?" he demanded. "While you, who have the responsibility of the people in your care, have a glorious opportunity for saving money for your corporation by conserving working efficiency through the prevention of focal infections . . . you shall be held in large part responsible for not only the physical efficiency but for the morbidity and tenure of life as well."[7]

Partly at Hyatt's and Price's urging, major employers including Armour & Co., H. J. Heinz, John Wanamaker, Kimberly-Clark, B. F. Goodrich, Sears Roebuck & Co., Macy's, Montgomery Ward, Lord & Taylor, International Harvester, and Colgate established dental clinics for their employees in the 1910s and 1920s.[8] "It has been my experience that ninety-nine percent of the employees of a large business house need both . . . examination and instruction," one dentist who participated in an industrial dental clinic program wrote, "and . . . only two out of seven thousand cases objected to what they called an infringement of their personal rights, when called upon to be examined."[9]

Even those who subscribed to the dental version of welfare capitalism, however, emphasized the importance of communicating to patients the value of individual effort, and of preserving for local dentists the opportunity to succeed in private practice. "The writer does not believe," one such proponent of the industrial hygiene clinic chided, "that under any consideration should a system be inaugurated which would give dental services absolutely free of charge. The financial expenditure for dental work received is an added incentive to better care of the mouth in the future, while anything which is given free is considered to be of little or no value."[10] Many companies offering dental services to their employees provided limited care, as at the Heinz Company, where "when more elaborate work is required, the patient is advised to consult outside dentists."[11] Other programs, like school hygiene clinics, offered only cleaning and examination, and similarly referred patients to

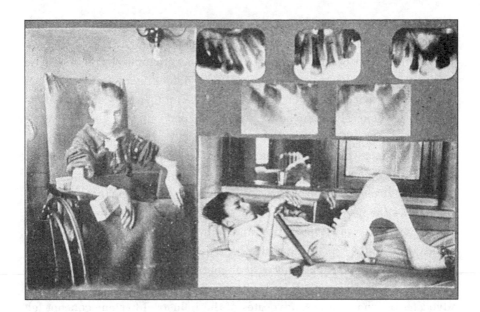

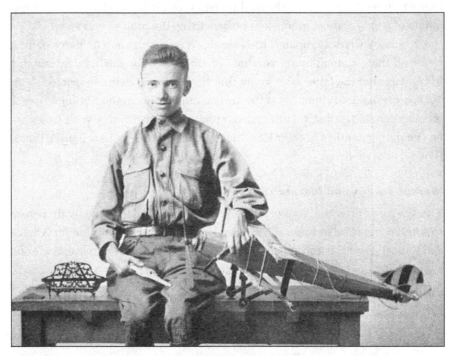

Figure 6 Before and after treatment for arthritis caused by dental infection. This image illustrated Weston Price's address to industrial managers on the benefits of employee dental hygiene programs. *Dental Items of Interest* 47 (December 1925): 890.

private dentists for restorative treatment. A few allowed employees to visit company dentists on company time, but at the employees' own expense.

Dentists who promoted industrial hygiene programs were careful to point out that, particularly in programs that did not provide restorative dental care, the provision of dental education and training in self-care helped the employees who received it to better understand and value the dental services they would seek out privately. This was, they felt, an advantage to the community dentists who provided the additional care. "The patient presents a clean, healthy mouth for his own dentist to work in," wrote the director of the Armour & Co. dental clinic in 1920, "and the dentist, realizing that his patient appreciates the necessity and value of the work to be done, approaches his task in a much more sympathetic frame of mind that [sic] is the case where he has to do all the explaining himself and at the same time sell a bill of dentistry to the prospective patient with a mouthful of bad teeth that are painful, diseased, and very often foul with heavy deposits of tartar."[12] Like the advocates of school clinics, advocates of the industrial hygiene concept felt that a proliferation of well-informed patients would help to hasten the retirements of poorly trained practitioners, benefiting the profession as a whole. At the Kimberly-Clark Company, in Neenah, Wisconsin, the company dentist reported that "a much better service is being given by outside dentists due to the fact that the latter now know that their work is being inspected."[13] In 1918, a speaker told attendees at the annual convention of the National Dental Association that industrial clinic programs "[tend] to do away with bad work on the part of dentists in their localities, because those dentists realize that if they wish to retain their clientele they must do better work."[14]

Market Forces and Market Disruptions

The system of private dental practice, generously supplemented by dispensaries and school and industrial hygiene clinics, sufficed to provide for Americans' most urgent dental needs through the 1920s. But the massive market failures and the terrible privation of the Depression posed new challenges to dentists' insistence that the private market, combined with the availability of charity care, could do enough for Americans' dental health. American dentists recognized that many people required dental services for which they were unable to pay. Furthermore, they acknowledged that their own attempts to limit entry to the profession had resulted in a shortage of dentists, which particularly affected rural areas of the United States and which reflected badly on the profession as a whole. Their suggestions about how to remediate these problems emphasized the voluntary, the temporary, and—whenever possible—programs paid for by someone other than the government.

Physicians, too, faced the accusation that their monopoly on health services placed crucial health care out of Americans' reach. Because of the same market pressures, New Dealers were intensely interested in creating a program for the socialization of health care costs in the United States. By 1935, the Roosevelt administration's Committee on Economic Security described health insurance as "the most immediately practicable and financially possible form of economic security."[15] The reaction of American physicians to New Deal–era proposals for national health insurance was swift and direct. Denouncing compulsory insurance plans as socialist, the American Medical Association objected even to voluntary plans on the grounds that they often served as a route to compulsory, perhaps government-subsidized, insurance. Attempts to appeal to the financial interest of physicians by emphasizing the potentially income-stabilizing effects of health insurance failed dismally with an audience that, for the most part, no longer feared personal financial instability. As the Depression worsened, and demand for medical care fell, the AMA began to accept the idea that voluntary health insurance plans could be advantageous for both physicians and patients.[16] But the AMA's opposition to compulsory insurance plans—and particularly for those administered by the government—remained vigorous.

Many dentists had similar misgivings about the prospect of insurance. As with physicians, however, their initial distaste for all plans of third-party payment was softened somewhat by the economic instability they experienced during the Depression. Dentists had long believed that working-class Americans undervalued dental services, but the Depression placed dental care out of the financial reach of even those who had been able to afford it, and who had actively sought it in the past. The stopgap of the industrial dental clinic failed, as millions of Americans were thrown out of work and out of proximity to such programs. "Today it is not the poor child who is always with us," wrote A. C. Wherry, the president-elect of the ADA, in 1933, "but it is the boy and the girl from the average home whose parents yesterday were classed as the esteemed patients of our average dental office, who is deprived of dental care."[17] Wherry argued that the cumulative nature of dental impairment, which would persist long after the economic contraction that had caused it, made dentists' commitment to get Americans through the Depression with healthy teeth particularly important. Failure would mean that Americans suffered worse dental health for decades to come. And the increasing prevalence of untreated dental decay made dentists look bad: in the New Deal era, opposition to even comparatively drastic programs for the distribution of vital resources could be construed as opposition to the reinvigoration of the catastrophically failed American economy.

Patient demand for dental services lay, tantalizingly, just beyond dentists' reach. Everywhere they turned—in popular magazines, advertisements, and the movies—dentists were reminded that Americans maintained an active interest in health care interventions promising improvements in personal appearance. The idea that an "inferiority complex" about appearance might impede a person's success in both public and private life carried particular currency for Americans continually encountering the economic catastrophes of the 1930s and early 1940s. One way to improve one's outlook and thereby retake control of one's personal fortunes, this theory suggested, was to work on one's external physical qualities. The new ethos that resulted manifested itself not only in Americans' interest in dentistry, but in plastic surgery and in the culture of "personal improvement" that sprang up in the form of exercise fads, pop psychology, and Americans' heightened concern about the appearance of their teeth.[18]

Personal-care product manufacturers aggressively promoted the idea that having a pleasant mouth was critically important to one's social and psychological success, and receptive Americans flocked to purchase products intended to enhance their attractiveness. Listerine advertisements, for example, simultaneously reflected and created the fear that aesthetic flaws might have social consequences. In a June 1930 ad published in *Good Housekeeping*, a stylish young woman stared bleakly into her empty dance card. She was surrounded by the comments she had overheard from fellow dancegoers: "They never invite her twice," "She's a nice girl, but—" "Has she always been that way?" and, more ominously, "I don't blame him for breaking the engagement," and "She simply cannot hold onto a fellow."[19] The text below the graphics read: "Halitosis (unpleasant breath) is too high a hurdle for sensitive people. You yourself cannot be sure that at this very moment you are free of halitosis. . . . The swift, certain way to put your breath beyond suspicion is to rinse your mouth with full strength Listerine."[20] Fresh breath, the ad suggested, was important to the self-confidence and social success that eluded so many Americans during the Depression.

Dentists helped to keep Americans' underlying interest in dentistry high by promoting it as a salve for all manner of personal and national ills. Popular literature and short films aimed at American youth advertised orthodontics, increasingly facilitated by war-era improvements in materials science, as a way to ensure social success. The social benefits of orthodontics were typically presented in a fashion that balanced them judiciously with other health concerns, but it was clear to patients that they could expect great social results from their time in the dental chair. For example, after the protagonist's visit to the orthodontist in *Betty's Crooked Teeth* (circa 1937), her teacher said "Betty, your schoolwork is improving. Last year your average was N minus, now it is S." The school nurse, too, had good news: "Betty, you have gained in weight, your health is better." At the end of the film, the narrator announced that "Betty's straight teeth will increase her self-confidence as she grows older. Straight teeth aid in developing a pleasing appearance, expression and personality, in business and social life." The film cut to one example of the powerful effect of straight teeth—in the person of the orthodontist's receptionist, a welcoming young woman with a brilliant—and straight—smile.[21] Such presentations of the benefits of dentistry were calculated to appeal to Americans seeking ways of taking firmer control of their personal fortunes, but they also helped to keep patients' underlying interest in dental care high.

Socializing Dental Costs

It was not an absolute decline in demand, but the gap between patients' desire for service and their ability to pay, that so bedeviled dentists who faced declining business in the 1930s and 1940s. The possibility of closing this gap prompted a few dentists to seriously propose the socialization of dental care in the early 1930s. Their first concern was for children: many dentists pointed out the curious discrepancy between Americans' acceptance of socialized education and their rejection of socialized medical and dental service. "Why does it pauperize a child to give it health service and not when giving it education?" demanded the editors of the *Journal of the Michigan State Dental Society*.[22] Ever-mindful of contemporary arguments for economy, they pressed the claim that "education that does not include health service is wasteful, for education depends for its usefulness on health . . . the present method of prodigality in education and parsimony in health service is untenable."[23] Others noted that the socialization of education had improved the status of teaching as a profession and the literacy of the population as a whole, suggesting that dentists and the broader American public could hope for similar outcomes from socialized health and dental care.[24]

The example of the military provided a ready reference for those who argued that socializing health care could work in the United States. During and after World War I, highly trained physicians and dentists provided care to American troops under the administration of a centralized command. A quasi-military system would eliminate patients' ability to choose their care providers, these advocates admitted—but then, "is it not a fact that the selecting of a doctor has for years been denied those charity patients who have availed themselves of the advantages of the larger, better-organized hospitals where scientific medicine has prevailed? . . . Today this freedom to choose a doctor may actually redound to the disadvantage of the patient not knowing where to procure the best advice."[25] The military system was also an advantage for dentists, they argued, because it provided income stability and better living conditions than the vagaries of private practice. "Physicians and dentists work at definite yearly salaries, are amply provided with food, shelter, and clothing, a home and maid service—and retire at night with greater mental calm, awake at reveille to face more sunshine than comes into the lives of our glorified individualists in private practice."[26] A military system of employment for dentists would, they felt, cost less per capita than the existing hodgepodge of private, charity, industrial and school care. " 'We have found an army post at Fort Benning, Georgia, spending thirty-five dollars per capita for a service which in most respects seems ideal in quality.' Is this not enough testimony for the necessity of completely socializing medicine upon a naval or military foundation?" one demanded.[27] Directing a barb at the American Medical Association's claim that government-funded health care removed individual practitioners' incentives for professional excellence, proponents of a military system pointed out that the AMA had admitted to membership "every medical officer in the navy and army" for more than twenty-six years.[28]

More frequently, however, those who argued for socialization of American dentistry gestured not towards the military but toward other countries to illustrate the benefits of socialized health and dental care. "We have but to look beyond the borders of our country to find about twenty countries with medicine in varying states of stages of socialization," one writer mused.[29] Such writers debated whether compulsory social insurance, to which they sometimes referred as "partial socialization," or the direct employment of dentists by government, or "full socialization," would be preferable. They generally agreed that the inaccessibility of dental care in the Depression-era United States contrasted poorly with the free availability of a basic standard of dental treatment in countries with either fully or partially socialized medicine and dentistry. Health outcomes were better when medicine was socialized, they argued, and the opportunities for malfeasance by unscrupulous or inept physicians and dentists were reduced.

Comparison to conditions of health and dental care elsewhere immediately opened the rhetorical door to reminders of the deficiencies of British dentistry, and—more frequently and pervasively—to the defects of the Soviet system of socialized medicine and dentistry. Reference to dental practice in Russia, like other examples of dental practice abroad, had long provided a way for American dentists to discuss their hopes and fears about their professional status. As early as 1919, James H. Howell of the Michigan State Dental Society reported, in a comment that damned through faint praise, that "as good, if not better, dentistry is seen in Russia as I have seen done in our sister country, England."[30] American dentists credited the ministrations of professional dentists with helping to stem the tide of political radicalism at home: the journal *Oral Hygiene* reported "one of London's leading men in the dental world" as saying that he had "never seen a Bolshevist with other than bad teeth. Proper care of the teeth obviates the mental explosions that cause Bolshevism."[31] They hoped that the presence of a small group of professional dentists in Russia might help to, as the writer of one caption to an image of a Russian peasant being attended to by a dentist put it, "'restrain' the Bolsheviki."[32] But by the 1930s, as Communist party rule in the Soviet Union hardened, it was clear to American dentists that dental care in the USSR had gone horribly wrong. "One hasty glance into the mouth of any person coming to us from any country in the world which 'enjoys' state or insurance dentistry is all a dentist needs to determine its 'blessings,'" a Los Angeles dentist wrote in 1933. "So, before we allow our people to be propagandized into once more following Europe's lead into disaster, let the American dental profession once more take the lead . . . by solving conclusively this vexed problem as to how to make the necessity for dentistry plain to every worthy member of society."[33]

Soviet dentists argued—often in the pages of American dental journals— that the socialization of dental care had improved both the state of the profession and Soviet citizens' dental health. In 1929, I. A. Gershanski, a dentist from Odessa, commented that "during the reign of czardom, dentistry was in a state of extreme debasement in Russia. . . . At the present time, the profession of the dentist in Russia is delivered from the yoke of serfdom."[34] Gershanski was emphatic about the positive impact of categorizing dentistry as a branch of medicine, and requiring medical training of prospective dentists—a move that many American dentists opposed, but which had the advantage of promising to elevate the public image of dentistry. However, Gershanski spent the largest portion of his article describing the institutions of state dentistry in Russia, where more than 60 percent of ten thousand dentists were government employees and where, as he wrote approvingly, "Private dental practice is small and is steadily decreasing year by year."[35] Gershanski argued that nationalization of dental care had raised the professional status and quality of life of Russian dentists, who worked an average of five hours per day.[36] Reports emphasizing the positive health impact of these changes were also common: in 1930, Leningrad dentist George Randorf observed that the percentage of carious teeth in the mouths of Odessa children had decreased from between 72–95 percent before the Revolution to 5–8.6 percent after. "Surely," he wrote, "this comparatively small percentage of carious teeth of the children of the post-Revolution period must be due largely to the more satisfactory health of the mouth cavity and the modern prophylactic measures, which, as some of the actual aspects of social dental treatment, contribute to the decrease of the development of caries."[37] Randorf, too, regarded the state's assumption of responsibility for the provision of dental care as a positive move, and he hoped that his readers would agree.

American dentists, however, expressed hesitation about any system of paying for dental treatment that removed dentists from the stimulating rigor of direct engagement in commerce. Reflecting on the incorporation of dental care into the national health program of Britain, for example, New York dentist Solomon Gross wrote that "the entrance of a cold impersonal third party into the relations between dentist and patient has had a deadening effect upon the professional ardor and zeal of the members of the profession."[38] A 1932 item in the *Dental Digest*, addressing frequently asked questions about dentistry in the Soviet Union, devoted several inches of column space to answering the question "What stimulus is there for a dentist to work under the Soviet System?" The respondent, native Chicagoan Peter Swanish, answered that "one can live with less anxiety and fear as a state dentist than as a private practitioner."[39] Swanish considered the diminution of anxiety that came with state-controlled practice a bad sign: he believed that it marked a dangerous subversion of the healthy anxiety of the profit motive.

Swanish's interest in the systemic encouragement or discouragement of work in the Soviet Union mirrored the concern of American dentists about the existence of such incentives or disincentives in other national economies. In studying the USSR, rather than citing the influences of climate or genetic inheritance, they placed blame for the discouragement of work exclusively on the Soviet economic system. Though they believed that "real Americans" could be identified partly by their avid commitment to work, they feared providing un-American slackers with any temptation to shirk labor. Therefore, many Americans—including many dentists—believed that the American economic system had to be arranged so as to continually inspire Americans' productive efforts. Socialized medical and dental care would, they felt, "substitute for the will to get well and the will to work, the will to stay sick and the will to loaf."[40] The African American dentists of the National Dental Association took a less pessimistic view, counseling that American innovation could produce a system of socialized health care that would protect the impetus to work: "We do not anticipate an imitation of either the Soviet or the British pattern . . . [we promote a] form adopted to our American needs and democratic way of life," one black dentist wrote.[41] The notoriety of poor dental care in the British and Soviet systems of socialized medicine was a serious psychological obstacle for other American dentists. One Chicago writer urged his peers to observe carefully the results of socialized care in those locations, speculating in January 1933 that if Americans could successfully "stave off these schemes for another ten years, we will be spared them, because they will prove to be so harmful to medical practice and so destructive to national character that we will escape their blight."[42]

Meeting the Demands of War

The ten years that followed the New Deal brought complications that dentists hoping for the opportunity to recover from the Depression and return to normal life could barely have imagined. Chief among them were a startling increase in demand for dental care, accompanied by a precipitous decline in the national supply of dentists. The wartime economic boom increased Americans' disposable incomes, and restrictions placed on many commodities helped to direct consumer spending towards other goods and services—and especially toward dental care. "Women who never did a thing but go to card parties and take care of their homes, are now working in war industries of the nation drawing weekly wages that run from fifty dollars up to incredibly high sums," warned one California dentist. "Most of these people put off their dentistry during the depression years. Now, with inflated wages, they are crowding the dental offices of our country. Dentistry is one service the government hasn't restricted."[43]

Dentists contributed to the war effort by encouraging young men and women to become dentally "fit to fight." In 1944, for example, a skit promoting "A War Angle in Dental Health Teaching" emphasized the national-security ramifications of dental decay, giving a "happy-looking" Hitler these nefarious lines: "My spies tell me that the American school children don't want good teeth. That pleases me. I want all American school girls and boys to have bad teeth. Then we'd conquer them without a shot. . . . You see those boys and girls have turned against their flag and are helping me, the great Hitler. . . . We'll conquer America because the children don't care." The skit recommended that children avoid spending money on candy and movies and purchase war stamps and bonds instead, or that they "have a parade with banners saying we're going to have good teeth to chew Hitler to pieces."[44]

These blandishments about dentistry stimulated patient demand for dental services that were already scarce. According to a survey sponsored by the office of the Surgeon General in 1943, more than half of all dentists under the age of thirty-five served in the military during World War II, leaving a dangerous shortage of practitioners at home. Though those who remained stateside increased their efforts, there were simply not enough dentists to meet Americans' rising demands for dental care. The resultant shortfall between demand and supply left many Americans with the impression that the dental profession could not be relied upon to consider national needs above individual pecuniary interests.

Dentists recognized that Americans' alienation from the system of private-practice dentistry boded badly for the future of their profession. During the war years, they debated a variety of measures for increasing the availability of quality dental service. Some—like the suggestion that dentists increase their night office hours and focus their work on the adolescents who might soon be marching off to war—caused little controversy.[45] Other plans touched on more closely held facets of dentists' professional self-concept, and drew much more opposition. One faction, led by New York dentist Charles Hyser and Claude Pepper, the US senator from Florida, promoted a renewed consideration of the "level-technician" plan in which a small cadre of highly educated dentists supervised the work of a larger group of lesser-trained service providers. Opponents of the plan protested that it would damage the unity of the profession and subject Americans to poor-quality care. "The so-called 'Hyser Plan,'" thundered Alfred Asgis, a faculty member at the New York University College of Dentistry, "is a dismemberment plan of dentistry. . . . It is our obligation to those who will return from the field of battle to provide them with high quality dental service," not the ministrations of lesser-trained assistants.[46] Some stateside military dentists began sending patients who needed relatively uncomplicated prosthetic work directly to dental laboratories to be fitted for dentures and partial plates. "Such detestable practice has too many complications for comfort," retorted the editor of the *Texas Dental Journal.* "However, such is being forced upon [the laboratories] by unthinking members of the profession," who failed to appreciate the importance of dentists' professional control over all phases of dental service.[47] New Jersey dentists reconsidered legislation allowing dental hygienists to practice without dentists' supervision, though they ultimately rejected the idea of permitting hygienists to "compete with the ethical dentist who has spent years and thousands of dollars in an effort to be competent and maintain a professional high standing."[48]

Dentists from many locales complained that the lack of reciprocity in state licensing laws restricted their ability to move to the places where more dentists were needed: these laws, they felt, reflected the unseemly interest of state dental society leaders in ensuring their personal fortunes at the expense of others. "It is high time the public was rescued from the clutches of a few 'closed shop' dentists who prate of dental standards. . . . If we had full and nation-wide reciprocity in the dental profession, there would be a more equal distribution of dentists throughout the country," one argued, *"There would be less demand for socialized dentistry."*[49] In a similar vein, the editors of *Dental Survey* urged willing dentists to consider establishing practices in rural areas that lacked dentists. "Shortage of dentists, bad distribution of dentists—those are the explosion caps that can set off the powder of demands for socialization legislation," the writers warned. Indeed, they suggested, dentists' own efforts to disseminate dental health education had only made the problem more acute, since Americans who knew the facts about the need for regular dental care "feel their lack more keenly."[50]

African American dentists, who treated some of the most underserved patients in the United States, shared the sense that the socialization of health and dental care costs would be a positive good. There was roughly 1 dentist per 7,000 black Americans in 1930, and 1 per every 9,000 in 1940.[51] Dentists and patients alike suffered because of the discrepancy between the amount of care needed and the availability of money and manpower to provide it. Black Americans' continued experience of domestic racism cloaked in arguments for regional and local uniqueness also helped to persuade them of the importance of intervention that occurred at the federal level. As a result, the National Dental Association generally favored plans for federally provided health and dental insurance. "We cannot stop a trend so well founded upon public needs when the public is aroused," the editors of the *Bulletin of the National Dental Association* counseled.[52]

The American Dental Association, however, was desperate to avoid solutions imposed from without: the number and diversity of plans dentists considered to remediate the dental manpower shortage highlighted this. One particularly eager Chicago dentist suggested that dentists "Look into This Unionism Business," as a means for fighting to retain—and even improve—dentists' professional prerogatives. He pointed out that "at present there is not one organized craft whose members do not receive more money than the dentists in our state and county institutions," and suggested that organizing into unions might provide dentists with the opportunity to command better pay.[53] Though his idea fell on unreceptive ears, it was clear to all observers that some change in the American system of health care distribution was in the offing. Dentists hoped to maintain as much control as possible over what happened to their profession, and when.

The Threat of Dental Insurance

As the Allied victory approached, and as calls for some form of national health insurance at home increased, most dentists came to accept the notion that insurance would play a permanent role in their professional practices. Dentists who treated low-income patients actually welcomed the idea, and urged their colleagues to act selflessly for the greater good. Addressing the commencement ceremony of Meharry Medical College in 1943, for example, Howard University Dental School Dean Dixon implored graduates: "Have you ever thought that you as the more fortunate members of a minority group enjoy a rare privilege—a privilege of reaching out and rendering an unrestricted good for the helpless and appreciative masses whose dependence upon you is like that of an innocent child, who looks to a parent with unfailing faith?"[54] Other dentists, with somewhat less public spirit, merely sought to head off more drastic proposals for state control of dental service by putting forward an agreeable plan that would insure a threshold level of dental care for all. Alfred Asgis, for instance, conceded that in addition to the traditional nostrums of providing for children's dental health, promoting additional dental health education and securing funding for advanced dental research, "compulsory social insurance on a national scale (with proper safeguards for quality and quantity of services) should be established as a social means of providing dental health care to the low income groups."[55] Asgis complained when initial Congressional attempts to enact national health care omitted provisions for dentistry, and recommended that fellow dentists write to the legislators involved to remind them of "the importance of quality dentistry."[56]

Unfortunately for the cause of Asgis's letter-writing campaign, however, most American dentists, like their physician counterparts, opposed Congress's postwar moves towards national health insurance legislation. Though its Congressional proponents had already seen their proposals for the expansion of Social Security's limited health programs defeated in two previous incarnations, the 1945 version of the Wagner-Murray-Dingell bill sought to capitalize on the pro-democracy rhetoric of the war era by again attempting to enact socially insured health coverage. Physicians campaigned furiously against the legislation, which they claimed would make them "slaves."[57] Similarly, seventy-seven percent of white dentists opposed the measure.[58] (Despite the resounding success of "slavery" rhetoric with white health professionals, the National Dental Association favored Wagner-Murray-Dingell.)

Dentists generally feared that dental insurance, whether voluntary or compulsory, would restrict their professional autonomy and eat into their profits. Then, too, they had sincere concerns about being asked to provide remedial dental care under any insurance plan to patients who had gone years—perhaps a lifetime—without dental treatment. "It would be like starting a new life insurance company that was to pay policies to the heirs of every man, woman and child who died in the last fifty years, and for whose insurance no premiums had been paid," one wrote.[59] Consistent with the increasingly strident anti-Communism of the postwar years, they also harbored more grandiose anxieties about the impact of socialized health expenditures on the American national character. One Iowa dentist projected that the Truman administration's health insurance plan would fail in fewer than five years because employees who were taxed for dental insurance would "grumble at slow service and for that reason many will quit their jobs rather than pay for something they are not getting."[60] Even the usually staid University of Michigan dental school professor Kenneth Easlick claimed that "a little social security, like a little morphine, may become habit forming," leading addled Americans to favor socialist policies for national health insurance. "The challenge to clear thinking, to unemotional scientific planning and to reasoning cooperation by dentists is obvious," he concluded.[61] In 1950, with bills for compulsory national health insurance again languishing in Congress, the president of the American Association of Orthodontists told a meeting of that organization that "compulsory health insurance, together with all other socialistic tendencies, will result in a further increase of autocratic power, granted to centralized government, to interfere in the private affairs of citizens and to regulate their daily lives, and will further curtail their freedom and liberty. . . . We should keep in mind that dental needs and service are, first of all, problems of the individual."[62]

Several independent forces helped to rescue American dentists from the horns of their postwar dilemma. Because of resounding physician opposition, and particularly because of the rising currency of arguments that opposed social insurance programs on the grounds of their similarity to Communism, Wagner-Murray-Dingell and similar plans were continually defeated in Congress. At the same time, labor unions made a tactical decision to support the growth of a private welfare state instead of public programs of social insurance: health benefits, unlike salary increases paid in cash, were not taxable, and both labor and management hoped that private insurance programs would command the loyalty of American workers. The voluntary insurance of health-care costs, including dental costs, surged in popularity, enhancing Americans' access to health care and relieving some of the pressure on Congress and the health professions to provide dental and health insurance.[63]

Dentists still hoped to convince a distrustful public that they had Americans' best interests at heart, and that the profession would not leave untreated patients in need of dental care. "The ultimate remedy" to the discrepancy between the supply of dentists and the demand for dentistry, the senior dental officer of the US Public Health Service wrote in 1944, "is the reduction of the dentists' patient-load through reduction of the incidence of dental disease. There is promise in that direction and much upon which to base our hopes. This statement is based on recent information on the prophylactic effects of the fluoride compounds."[64] In fluoride, dentists were on the verge of a discovery that would reduce the demand for reparative dental services, help keep dental costs within limits acceptable to the public, and provide dentists themselves with an opportunity to renew their images as the benevolent arbiters of modern, scientific dental research.

Chapter 5

Behind the Fluorine Curtain

Today, mid-twentieth century opposition to the fluoridation of public water supplies is widely remembered as the province of kooks. In Stanley Kubrick's 1964 post-nuclear classic *Dr. Strangelove, or: How I Learned to Stop Worrying and Love the Bomb*, General Jack D. Ripper, his name and character a caustic send-up of Vietnam-era anticommunist militarists, worried that "a foreign substance is introduced into our precious bodily fluids without the knowledge of the individual. Certainly without any choice. That's the way your hard-core Commie works." In the view suggested by Kubrick's portrayal of opposition to water fluoridation—and in the minds of many observers before and since—the addition of fluoride to Americans' drinking water was a self-evident good, opposed only by the irredeemably paranoid.

Dentists and many popular writers have portrayed water fluoridation as a necessary, welcome, and even inevitable step on the path toward late twentieth-century Americans' near-maniacal obsession with their teeth. In this view, fluoride was an obvious improvement to Americans' lives, and the fetishization of aesthetic interventions that followed it an inexorable result of Americans' improved dental health. This vision of the debate over fluoride, and what came after it, contains some grave errors. Its proponents have an incomplete view of dentists' motives for advocating water fluoridation—and of the basis for other Americans' opposition to it. More importantly, they ignore the ways in which the fight over fluoride helped dentists to view collective action for the public good with increasing skepticism, and thereby contributed to the rise of an individualist ethos about dental care at the end of the century.

Fluoride and Dental Aesthetics

Most twentieth-century hygiene campaigns portrayed good dental health and a pleasing facial appearance as critical to both individual achievement and the broader success of the American economy. From the outset, public and professional concern about the presence of fluoride in public drinking water hinged on this preexisting, active, and at times intense concern for the appearance of Americans' teeth. The first confirmed reports about the influence of chemical compounds in water on dental appearance came in 1925, when prominent New York dentist Frederick McKay described his travels to Benton, California, a town in the northern portion of the Mojave Desert, where users of water from the local hot spring developed brown mottling on their teeth. McKay felt certain that the hot springs were the source of the unsightly brown stain. Like most of his professional peers, he was already familiar with "Texas stain," an underdevelopment of the enamel associated with hard water, and eventually accompanied by a secondary brown, yellow, or pearly white mottling of the surface of the teeth. McKay's work in Benton was part of an emerging research project that would, within twenty years, identify the cause of the stain as an overabundance (more than one or two parts per million) of naturally occurring fluoride in the water supplies of areas where mottled enamel occurred.[1]

McKay reported that denizens of Benton, "a few scattered families on the adjacent ranches and a collection of Piute Indians on the hillside,"[2] had no other source of water. By way of contrast, he cited events in Oakley, Idaho, where dental mottling had led the local Women's Civic League to campaign for a bond referendum "from the proceeds of which the present source of water supply from the warm spring was to be discarded, and a new supply from a different source substituted."[3] McKay counted the situation as "the first instance where a policy of municipal economics of such magnitude as is involved in the abandonment of a water system and requiring a tax of the people, has been determined solely by and upon a dental aspect."[4] McKay pointed this out partly because it illustrated Idaho dentists' success at establishing themselves as authorities on science, and thus constituted a victory in dentists' ongoing campaign to raise the status of their profession. McKay had also been personally involved in spurring the passage of the bond referendum: "prominent and influential citizens" had argued that the link between the local water supply and dental mottling had not been clearly established, and McKay had addressed a town meeting the night before the

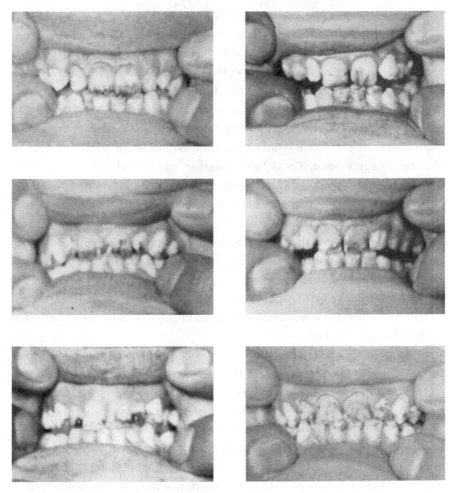

Figure 7 "Mottled enamel" as portrayed in Frederick McKay's 1925 article on fluoride. *Dental Cosmos* 67 (September 1925): 851.

election, "presenting the evidence which has been gathered during the past ten or more years . . . definitely connecting the water . . . with the existence of mottled enamel."[5]

McKay reported that the locals of Oakley, whom he described as both "citizens" and "taxpayers," "were convinced, after mature consideration of this fundamental and compelling point, that they had not the ethical right as parents and citizens to unload this blight upon the present generation of children of the community, nor upon generations yet unborn."[6] Oakley citizens' teeth were not more prone to decay or fall out as a result of the staining, but Oakleyites considered brown stains on their teeth a problem that required urgent attention, and this had a powerful impact on Oakley residents' thinking about what ought to be done about the town's water supply.

Mottled and stained enamel, they thought, was a blight on humanity. The best scientific explanation of the causative mechanism for mottled enamel suggested that it was too late to remediate the damage to adults' teeth. Generations to come, however, could be protected by the passage of the water supply bond. These facts, together with broader American sympathies for the protection of children, explained the locals' insistence on couching the bond issue in terms of their roles as parents. Their belief—and McKay's—that citizenship could and should play a role in the debate is more tantalizing. Oakleyites thought of the bond issue as a matter of citizenship partly because it was citizenship that conferred upon them the right to vote. They also imagined that there was something about the particular nature of the damage done by the local water that had bearing on the question of citizenship—that there was some way in which good-looking teeth and good citizenship were linked.

The class and regional dynamics of the mottled enamel problem, which primarily afflicted communities in the American West, played a role in this conviction. McKay concluded that the citizens of Oakley were to be praised for having "spared [future generations] the disfiguring appearance of this blight . . . [which] would advertise to the world that such persons were the products of a given community."[7] Most naturally fluoridated water supplies— almost eighty percent by the estimate of the American Dental Association's Bureau of Public Relations in 1943[8]—were in the West, a place where recent American immigrants frequently traveled to slip the bonds of their existing class and racial status. McKay alluded gently to the widespread popular suspicion that the Americans who populated the rural and hardscrabble West had something to hide about their backgrounds. Rural Westerners who attempted integration into American city life might, he thought, find themselves marked by their mottled teeth and therefore socially handicapped by the visible evidence of their geographic origins. Like immigrants, Americans from the rural West faced the real prospect of reduced class mobility because of their failure to conform to the increasingly shared image of what Americans' teeth should look like.

The US Public Health Service quickly developed an interest in finding out what was causing mottled enamel—and in eliminating whatever the offending factor might be.[9] In the early 1930s, dental surgeon H. Trendley Dean traveled extensively under the auspices of the US Public Health Service, investigating the connections between cases of "mottled enamel" in children and the existence of fluorospar mines (in this period, usually operated by the Aluminum Corporation of America) near those children's water supplies.

The rapidity and expansiveness of the federal government's expression of concern proceeded partly from contemporary attempts to establish a clear field of endeavor for dentists—of similar influence and prestige to the position held by physicians—in the Public Health Service. In 1927, Senior Dental Surgeon C. T. Messner wrote an eight-page missive to Surgeon General Hugh Cumming, arguing for the organization of an independent Dental Section of the PHS. Messner felt that the new structure was necessary because "the field is so broad for this sort of work, and the possibilities of its expansion so great, that it can justify a section to itself, and in this way will be able to render service to the limits of its appropriation, which might not be the case were it tied with other interests equally as important."[10] Messner's correspondence repeatedly referenced the deplorable state of American children's dental health, usually focusing on the functional losses that resulted. Messner did also point out that the loss of a first permanent molar could create "a deformity of the face and cranium," which suggests that aesthetic concerns were not absent—though, meriting only one line of an eight-page single-spaced letter, neither were they prominent.

However, the first target of the new dental section of the Public Health Service was not a functional but an aesthetic concern. Despite the occasionally shocking appearance of teeth damaged by an excess of naturally occurring fluoride, the mottled enamel problem was strictly aesthetic—most teeth affected by the presence of natural fluoride in water supplies were stronger and more resistant to decay than teeth that had not been exposed to fluoride during the critical childhood years, when the enamel of permanent teeth was forming. As one writer pointed out, reflecting in 1965 on the early history of fluoridation research, "It was a hope to improve an undesirable appearance that prompted Black [another early researcher] and McKay, and later Dean, to study the relationship between fluorides in drinking water supplies and a condition termed 'mottled enamel.'"[11] The federal government's interest in the problem of mottled enamel was not an inevitable outgrowth of the Public Health Service's interest in dental health, narrowly defined as the preservation of functional dentition. Public Health Service officers like H. Trendley Dean studied the problem of mottled enamel because the federal government considered the "blight" that stained Americans' teeth a matter of national concern all by itself.

The discovery of fluoride compounds as the cause of both mottled enamel and improved resistance to decay led a decades-long debate over the propriety of artificially fluoridating public water supplies. The Bureau of Public Relations of the American Dental Association reported in 1943 that "the continuous use throughout the formative period of the tooth of water containing about 1 part per million of fluorine will result in an incidence of approximately 10 per cent of the mildest forms of dental fluorosis. Thus, the logical approach from a public health standpoint to the prevention of this disease is the avoidance of the use of domestic water containing fluorine much in excess of this amount. . . . Reduction of the fluoride content, however, much below 1 part per million of fluorine may not be advisable, in view of the recent epidemiologic evidence concerning the low dental caries experience rates associated with the use of domestic water containing this approximate fluoride concentration."[12] Though the staining caused by excess fluoride was clearly unsightly, the strengthening of dental enamel caused by low concentrations of fluoride in drinking water struck dentists—and many laypeople—as highly desirable.

Accordingly, dentists began a locality-by-locality campaign for the fluoridation of public water supplies at appropriate levels. During these years, both advocates and detractors of the practice made frequent, and contradictory, reference to the aesthetic effects of fluoride on human teeth. The development of an unambiguous aesthetic justification for—or argument against—fluoridation was hampered from the outset by the fact that diagnosis of "mottled enamel" was sometimes a subtle one. Though high levels of naturally occurring fluoride could produce dark brown stains that no dentist (or layperson) could miss, lower levels of fluoride might produce no aesthetic changes, or only very subtle ones. H. Trendley Dean's correspondence with Surgeon General Hugh Cumming was rife with examples of reported cases which, upon investigation, proved to have been "mistaken for 'calcium deficiency spots' on the enamel surface of the teeth," and of towns in which "there were three or four cases which might be considered questionable, but not a single case where a diagnosis of even a mild type of mottled enamel could be made."[13]

The difficulty of diagnosing dental fluorosis was compounded by disagreement over whether all fluoride-mediated aesthetic changes to the teeth were bad changes. Most American dentists and dental researchers claimed that at the low level at which public water supplies would be fluoridated, mottled enamel would be of little, if any, concern. One author reported in 1966 that "the only proven detriment of fluoridation that may occur is enamel mottling (It has not occurred with any degree of consistency). The degree of mottling is extremely variable and is purely an esthetic disadvantage, showing no harmful effects on the tooth structure itself. Against this is to be placed a mass of evidence gathered by the American Dental Association . . . showing conclusively that the incidence of dental caries can be reduced by up to 60 per cent by a controlled program of water fluoridation. The scales do not balance."[14] Some writers acknowledged the possible occurrence of mottled enamel, but claimed that it was "generally not an esthetic problem"; whether they claimed this because it appeared infrequently or because, in its milder forms, some experts actually considered it an aesthetic advantage is unclear.[15] A few writers did explicitly try to turn the likelihood of dental fluorosis into an asset by claiming that mild fluorosis enhanced, rather than diminished, one's appearance. "The milder forms of fluorosis produce a tooth enamel with a high luster which enhances the beauty of teeth rather than disfigures them," claimed David Ast, New York State Director of Dental Health, in 1957.[16]

The most vigorous advocates of water fluoridation portrayed its aesthetic benefits to individuals as virtually unlimited. Beyond its effects on the enamel of the teeth, they felt, fluoride could prevent tooth loss, which occasioned aesthetic, social, and financial problems of its own. Partisans of fluoride argued that more decay-resistant teeth stayed in the mouth more reliably and made their possessors more attractive people. Most studies claimed a 60 to 65 percent reduction in dental caries as a result of "optimal" water fluoridation. An item from a Detroit-area newspaper of the 1960s summarized the pro-fluoride stance: "'Fluoridated water results in the formation of beautiful white teeth highly resistant to decay. . . . Speech defects, facial deformities, crooked teeth, disfigurement and pain, all result from dental decay."[17] During debate over a proposed 1963 antifluoridation legislative measure to require a popular vote before water fluoridation could occur in Detroit, speakers against the proposal included Kalamazoo pediatrician Frederick Margolis, who reported that the "change in children's teeth since the city's water supply had been fluoridated had been 'simply fantastic—they're beautiful.'"[18]

The aim of looking beautiful was widely understood to have freestanding merit. Dentists, in particular, increasingly considered Americans' loyalty to the goal of personal comeliness as an important adjunct to their efforts to insist on individual responsibility—and not dependence on a caretaker state—as the wellspring of American greatness. Consistent with this view, dentists who advocated water fluoridation frequently attempted to quantify the specific cash advantages of being better-looking. The director of the Michigan Department of Public Health, explaining to the state's Pure Water Council why the department advocated fluoride supplementation, argued that, with water fluoridation, "Not only is a more resistant tooth developed, but also a better appearing tooth is formed. . . . Decayed teeth may lead to disability and deformity. An aching tooth and a swollen face demolish the sense of mental, social and physical well being. The consequences of tooth decay can deter an individual from gainful pursuit or effective performance in earning a living."[19] Supporters of fluoridation in Detroit linked good dental health and freedom from pain with success at school and in work, but they also highlighted the importance of having a good-looking mouth to social acceptance and, thereby, to economic success. "Dental decay is painful, disfiguring, causes absenteeism from school and can prevent job placement and procurement," proclaimed the members of the Health Subcommittee of the Mayor's Committee for Total Action Against Poverty in 1965. The subcommittee voted to support fluoridation of public water supplies in Detroit.

Despite their reputation for obsessive interest in the political and environmental consequences of water fluoridation, antifluoridationists were also gravely concerned about the aesthetic impact of water fluoridation on Americans' teeth. Their aesthetic objections to even "optimal" levels of water fluoridation occurred early in public debates about fluoride, and were remarkably persistent. In fact, because the question of whether or not mild fluorosis was ugly was largely a matter of aesthetic preference rather than scientific judgment, the specter of bad-looking teeth was one of the most powerful arguments against fluoridation. Curiously, antifluoridation tracts usually did not include photographs of teeth affected by fluorosis: readers were left to imagine for themselves just how bad the problem could get. They were also encouraged to regard the debate among dentists about whether or not fluorosis was ugly as evidence of incompetence and perfidy. An item in the *National Fluoridation News*, an antifluoridation newspaper, reported that fluoridationists had first argued that no aesthetic change to the teeth would be wrought by fluoride supplementation: "Later, when first reported in Newburgh, NY, the fluoridationists cried, 'no disfiguring mottling can occur!' It has finally evolved promotionally that mottling in the test cities is now declared a 'cosmetic enhancement' making the teeth 'more beautiful.'"[20] Another flyer barked: "The P.H.S. expected and now reports mottling (white spots which may gradually become ugly brown or black stains) in the experimental town of Newburgh, N.Y. Health officers call these teeth 'beautiful.'"[21]

Like those who advocated for fluoride, antifluoridationists saw the effects of aesthetic damage to one's appearance as long-lasting and potentially quite severe. One antifluoridationist appealed to readers' sympathy for a girl who had been crippled by "fluorosis" (which the writer viewed as a full-body disease rather than as localized damage to tooth enamel): "Jennifer is a good looking girl with above average intelligence, but she is suffering from a disease that will not only affect her physically, but could very well submerge an already-shy personality. Jennifer has fluorosis. . . . Those of us in the neighborhood who have children with fluorosis are torn between the urge to show everyone the damage fluoride can do, and the desire to spare the children's feelings by not asking them to show their diseased teeth to the world." Another wrote: "Young girls are very conscious of their appearance, and disfigured teeth will give them feelings of inferiority that will remain with them all their lives. . . . It is pitiful that the poor little children must drink fluoridated water and bear this disfigurement and embarrassment while water works officials, such as in Newburgh, New York, have their own non-fluoridated artesian wells."[22] The linkage between dental appearance and psychological health seemed perfectly natural to these writers, and they expected it to seem just as natural to their readers.

Costs and Risks in the Fluoridation Debates

Partisans on both sides of the debate over the fluoridation of public water supplies agreed that Americans would want teeth that were healthy, intact, and free of unsightly stains. They differed in their aesthetic judgments about what was "unsightly," in their technical judgment about what would produce or protect against unsightliness, and, particularly, in their weighting of the costs involved to the public and the individual in achieving the aim of good teeth. It was this latter dispute that most clearly defined the ideological differences between the two groups.

Though dentists who advocated for fluoride hoped to use it in part to deflect demands for the socialization of health care costs, they understood that many Americans who were receptive to fluoride felt that way partly because of its potential to reduce overall health care expenditures. Therefore, they repeatedly emphasized the total dental savings that could be had for the low price of water supplementation: their research suggested that those savings were considerable. Studies of the two cities in New York State in which water had been first fluoridated in 1945 "established that dental costs are lower for children aged 6 and 7 years who have had fluoridated water all their lives. Initial dental care costs were $14.16 in Newburgh [the fluoridated city] and $32.38 in Kingston [the unfluoridated control]. Maintenance care the following year cost $5.90 in Newburgh against $11 in Kingston."[23]

Antifluoridationists, on the other hand, cited the high personal cost of remediating the damage done to human enamel by excessive, and sometimes even by "optimal," amounts of fluoride. Remediation of the severe staining that could accompany mottled enamel was possible: in 1942, two Arizona dentists reported that the use of a solution of superoxol (a 30% solution of hydrogen peroxide) and ether seemed to be effective against the stains that accumulated on mottled teeth, though it sometimes resulted in what one writer had referred to as a "ghastly" paper-white appearance.[24] Harold B. Younger, a Texas dentist, reported in the same year that the bleaching technique he advocated—one similar to the Arizona dentists'—would "be found to fill a long felt need for the relief of those cases to which it is particularly applicable and which otherwise must submit to tedious and annoying operative procedures, or go through life with disfiguring stains."[25]

Those who opposed water fluoridation usually shared dentists' commitment to the ideology of personal financial responsibility for health. More importantly, however, they prioritized avoiding negative health effects of government action over the danger of experiencing negative health effects from government inaction. They thus found the thought of having to pay individually for dental damage done by a public health program both economically undesirable and politically offensive. The Medical-Dental Committee on the Evaluation of Fluoridation, an antifluoridation organization, wrote: "Even if only one in 100 of the anticipated individuals suffers a severer degree of mottling, this will amount to about 200 such cases per 100,000 population, which is not insignificant either in terms of the number of individuals embarrassed by this affliction or the considerable dental costs entailed in attempting to correct it."[26]

Antifluoridationists sometimes positioned aesthetic damage as a mere index of less visible—but equally unacceptable—risk that they believed could be posed by the fluoridation of public water supplies. Because it was technically possible for high concentrations of fluoride to cause toxic effects in humans, many of fluoride's detractors considered it an environmental contaminant whose aesthetic effects at lower concentrations—however desirable on the surface—were properly regarded as evidence of pervasive harm. One antifluoridation organization pointed out that cows that consumed fluoridated water also developed mottled enamel, and that "a cow with mottled teeth is a poisoned cow, just as a child with mottled teeth is a poisoned child. Neither will ever be as well as if it hadn't happened."[27] Fluoride's opponents sometimes positioned their aesthetic claims as one of a concatenation of environmental, political, and medical arguments against fluoridation; a news item from 1963 included a ditty, allegedly sung to the tune of "Yankee Doodle": "Fluorides give you mottled teeth/ And they don't look so pretty/ They also clog up Mother Earth/ And make our water dirty."[28]

The choice to set these objections to the tune of a famous, almost instinctively recognizable patriotic song was a significant one. Participants in the fluoridation debates were not just arguing about the scientific and aesthetic wisdom of water fluoridation; they were also invoking a centuries-old dispute about the proper relationship between government authority and political liberty, between social systems and individual agency. The central domestic political issues of the 1960s raised the same questions in ways that helped to create a climate for a particularly bitter proxy fight over fluoride. What ought to be done for those left behind by American postwar prosperity? Would a "rising tide lift all boats," or would programs targeted to improve the condition of the poor be required—or justified? Would the poor "always be with us," or could a truly great society expect to eradicate poverty entirely? How could the interests of individuals and those of government and industry best be balanced?

During the peak years of the fluoridation debates, General Jack D. Ripper's certainty that Communists were out to "sap and impurify all of our precious bodily fluids" represented the belief, common on the political right, that large-scale state interventions intended to improve Americans' health could both literally and figuratively poison the body politic. Among Republicans and Southern Democrats, resistance to publicly funded programs for Americans' health and welfare was common, and helped to stymie congressional efforts to establish national health insurance.[29] Americans on the political right professed not to despise the poor themselves—in fact, they argued that their own resistance to state solutions helped to protect the interests of those most vulnerable to unintentional harm from "big government" programs like fluoride.

Concern about risks posed by government laxity or ineptitude existed on the political left as well. Leftist antifluoridationists charged that fluoridation was a plot orchestrated by aluminum companies to enable them to dispose of materials that would otherwise be considered toxic waste. In 1955, these accusations drove the Aluminum Company of America to issue a letter "deny[ing] that sodium fluoride is a waste product of aluminum manufacture" in order to combat such claims.[30] Because leftists were particularly attuned to the difficulty low-income Americans faced in evading threats without government assistance, concern about the risks fluoride posed to the poor continued to percolate in environmentalist circles.

The Nature of Citizenship and the Role of the State

Advocates of fluoridation argued that good teeth were critical to good citizenship. The public promotion of good dental health through the fluoridation of public water supplies would not only prevent individual suffering, they felt: it would also increase the percentage of Americans who were available to serve the nation's military and economic interests. The continued problem of finding draftees and volunteers for military service who were dentally fit to fight helped to shape these beliefs. As in World War I, the Second World War provided abundant example of the consequences of government inaction with respect to Americans' dental health. One writer reflected that "Even though the Armed Forces required that only six upper teeth make contact with six lower teeth, nearly 10 per cent of the men between 18 and 35 years of age did not qualify."[31] Accordingly, in 1943, a columnist in *Dental Health* magazine issued a "Challenge to High School Students," demanding: "Are you going to be one of the thousands of young people who, in the prime of their lives, cannot fulfill all the duties of citizenship because they neglected to make timely corrections of physical defects? What you do about correcting dental, eye, and other defects now, will be your answer to this challenge. It will be your answer to yourself, to your government, and to your future dependents."[32] The memory of negative answers to this challenge lingered in dental public health propaganda in favor of fluoride: "the largest cause for rejection of the first two million men examined in World War II," wrote one Detroit newspaper reporter in 1962, "was dental defects."[33]

By the 1960s, though, the rationale for the importance of good dental health had changed slightly. Actual physical ability to engage in combat lost significance. Much more important to fluoride's advocates was the symbolic success of the American economic system—particularly, in response to continued Communist claims to the contrary, in its ability to provide something approaching a fair chance of success for all. During Richard Nixon's 1959 debate with Nikita Khrushchev, the vice president taunted the Soviet premier with the claim that the American economic system made consumer goods like color televisions available to all who wanted them. Like Nixon, other adherents of the ideology of the liberal state hoped urgently for capitalism to create a "level playing field" such that communism and other forms of political radicalism would hold no appeal. Many Americans thus saw fluoridated water not only as an important public health reform, but as a way of demonstrating the fairness and equity of the American system itself.

This prompted interest in fluoridation from a wide range of individuals who were invested in the success of the American way of life. Particularly in cities notorious for their growing racial segregation, fluoride seemed like a way for government to evince the sort of benevolent interest in improving conditions that would head off more radical proposals for change. In 1963, for example, with Detroit's city budget in disarray, Juvenile Probate Court judge James H. Lincoln wrote to then-mayor Jerome P. Cavanaugh that "Taking the long view, fluoridation of the water supply will undoubtedly be the most important and far-reaching accomplishment during your administration. It is more important that the next generation have good teeth in the years to come than that Detroit have fiscal reform today."[34] Lincoln, who had served on the Detroit city council before becoming a juvenile court judge, wrote that "It would have been better to have delayed the Expressways, Cobo Hall, the Redevelopment programs, etc., for a few months and given the children of Detroit fluoridated water five or six years ago."[35]

In their arguments in favor of fluoridation, Detroit dentists, too, claimed that good teeth were an important part of good citizenship: "Dentists find it difficult to understand why some people would make second class citizens of their children by denying them good teeth through the simple, inexpensive and modern health procedure of water fluoridation," wrote fluoridation activist William Travis, a Detroit dentist who headed the Detroit District Dental Society's fluoridation campaign in the early 1960s, in a letter to the editor of a Detroit newspaper.[36] Travis, predictably, tried to position fluoridation as the scientific choice by referring to it as "modern" and stating that "dentists" could not understand why "some people" (i.e., not dentists) opposed it. He also argued that children who grew up without fluoridated water were, or would become, "second class citizens." The implication was twofold: bad dental health inevitably relegated one to "second-class status" not only because it was a sign that one's government disregarded one's suffering, but also because having unhealthy or ugly teeth had an impact on one's fitness for political participation. Dentists who advocated for fluoride cared deeply about this.

Opponents of water fluoridation worked from a very different understanding of the relative roles of the citizen and the state—and, relatedly, from
a different understanding of the proper relationship between individual and
public measures taken for the protection of health. They clearly feared the
threat of Communism to the American system—indeed, as Kubrick's film
portrayal of General Jack D. Ripper suggests, this was at times the most vivid
aspect of their arguments against fluoride. They argued that the highest value
of American politics was the protection of minority rights—and for them,
the minority to be protected could be as small as one. Good citizenship, in
this view, consisted in opposing measures that would jeopardize the rights
of individuals to be free from coercion, and specifically to avoid the deleterious physical and aesthetic effects of state-sponsored health programs. The
availability of a minimum standard of care to all was a far lower priority
than preventing the unwanted interference of the state in individual decisions about health.

Antifluoridationists—even laypeople—deployed the language of citizenship just as regularly and vehemently as did those who advocated for fluoride. When they used the word "citizen," however, they meant someone who
was entitled to protection from public-sector interference, and not someone
who could reasonably lay claim to the positive provision of a minimum standard of health. "I do not believe any citizen should have to drink water con-
taminated by a drug that is dangerous to health," wrote Mrs. McRouth, of
Detroit, to Mayor Cavanaugh in 1962.[37] Americans like McRouth pointed to
the unknown effects of fluoridated water on individuals with kidney disease,
diabetes, and allergies; many antifluoridationist materials cited the cases of
citizens who claimed to be allergic to elemental fluorine itself, and all of its
compounds, including those used for water fluoridation. "Even if one person
cannot take fluoride or object to having it in his drinking water *he should not
be forced to take it*," argued a 1965 pamphlet published by Detroit Citizens
Studying Fluoridation.[38] They viewed the fluoridation of public water supplies as a breach of the proper behavior of public health authorities, in which
public health powers could be exercised only when a contagious disease
threatened a larger population. They did not think that fluoridating water for
dental health was analogous to chlorinating it to kill infectious organisms:
they regarded chronic illnesses like dental decay, which they did not consider contagious, as inappropriate subjects of government intervention.

Notably, those who argued against fluoridation hewed to a commonly
held definition of citizenship that resolutely excluded children. Citizens were

those who could vote and were entitled to full autonomy over their bodies; public health programs benefiting those of whom that was not true were even more suspect. As the Detroit Citizens Studying Fluoridation pointed out, "no benefit [of fluoridation is] claimed to people over 10 years of age."[39] Even the most ardent fluoridationists did not believe that fluoride could improve adults' dental health; though some speculated that fluoride might lower the risk of osteoporosis in old age, research about this proved inconclusive. These facts emboldened antifluoridationists to deploy arguments highlighting the refusal rights of autonomous adult citizens at full force.

Compounding the antifluoridationists' arguments, those who advocated for fluoride failed to connect the fate of Detroit's children with the interests of the aged, thereby ceding some ideological ground in the war to define American citizenship. Dentist William Travis' belief that children could be even loosely described as citizens marked a distinctively profluoridation way of thinking about the public's responsibility to the young: typically, those who supported fluoride went out of their way to illustrate the long-term social benefits of investment in young people's health. Yet one of the major means of organizing voters to cast ballots in favor of fluoridation in Detroit was the dissemination of literature through the public schools. This tactic virtually ensured that older Detroiters would not only miss out on hearing a profluoridationist message, but could easily come to view fluoridation as a children's— and, therefore, not a citizens'—issue.[40]

Fluoridation-resistant American adults were particularly provoked by the invitation to view the interests of children as separate from, and sometimes in opposition to, their own. During the youth and adolescence of baby boomers, one could hardly fail to notice the presence of an unprecedented population of youth—the American landscape was literally rebuilt for their benefit, with construction of suburban homes and schools and other physical sites for young people surging during this period. The baby boom was accompanied by large new federal commitment of funds to programs for the elderly, but debate about Social Security and Medicare helped to persuade senior citizens that their interests hung tenuously in the balance, and that the aged couldn't afford the luxury of solidarity with the young. Backlash against the demographic transition thus helped to undergird arguments against public-sector health and welfare interventions, particularly when they were portrayed as beneficial to children.

Advocates on both sides of the fluoridation question exploited the tension that resulted. Skeptical Detroiters, for instance, were targeted for organizing on the basis of age: one pro-fluoride writer identified the anti-fluoride campaign there as "[preying] on the fears of the unsuspecting, the uninformed, and the elderly."[41] Similarly, a profluoridation dentist reported in a 1964 volume of the *Journal of the American Dental Association* that "it is the elderly who are concerned about the 'waste' of financing fluoridation for benefit of the young with possible ill effects on themselves."[42] In 1963, Mrs. Roy Percy, a resident of Detroit, sent Mayor Jerome Cavanaugh a pamphlet from the Ohio Pure Water Association, arguing that "One tenth of 1% of the water is consumed by children who may benefit from it. More than 99% of the tax money spent on fluoridation goes down the drain."[43] Mrs. Percy's accompanying letter read, in part: "I'm sure nobody is going to vote for the once [sic] that voted it in. I know so many on this street said the same thing. Clear our City Hall, the once that want to spin [sic] our money. Can't make ends meet now, with all the taxes we have to pay."[44] The public statements of health commissioners in fluoridated towns like New York City, who "lauded the [City Council's vote for fluoridation] as 'a priceless gift to the children and parents of New York City,'" didn't help: the question of who was paying for that gift was all too much on the minds of the older Americans who opposed fluoridation on financial grounds.[45]

Profluoridation publications, in reply, drew unflattering comparisons between the older public's receptivity to Medicare and their resistance to fluoridation. Advocates of fluoride attempted to convince voting adults of the need for fluoridation on economic grounds—whether or not the aged benefited personally from fluoride, dentists pointed out, their taxes would pay for either it or the much more expensive remedial dental care provided through publicly funded programs of dental care, which were under historic population strain. In so arguing, dentists only succeeded in more deeply ingraining the notion that taxation, the socialization of health care expenditures, and government as a whole profited the young at the expense of the old.

Those who advocated fluoridation and those who opposed it could not agree about whose needs ought to be regarded as compelling to the state. They also disagreed about what the state, even when compelling need existed, ought to be allowed to do. Yet every credible participant in political arguments about fluoride—and indeed, most fringe participants as well—agreed that Communism was a bad thing, and that there was an extreme of Communist-seeming "big government" that ought to be avoided. This belief was particularly strong among Southerners, who were already accustomed to thinking of states' rights as fundamental goods that were threatened by federal government action. The long-established tradition of local autonomy in American government—particularly with respect to public health measures like liquor laws, and the establishment of institutions, like schools, intended to benefit youth—resonated everywhere. Early in the efforts to fluoridate public water supplies, even most of those who favored fluoridation emphasized that it was politically and morally important for the decision to fluoridate water to be made locality by locality. "Such a decision must be made by public health officials and the public," opined one Wisconsin dentist, "It is important that the decision is made at the *local* level, not at the national level."[46] Dentists' commitment to this principle helped to assuage the fears of many Americans—even those who came down on the side of fluoridation—that the fluoridation of public water supplies would set off a "domino effect" transferring local power to "big government."

Nevertheless, water fluoridation proposals particularly irked those who were already embroiled in debates about state power and authority. In 1963, Houston attorney W. Hume Everett addressed that city's chapter of a dental fraternity on the topic of "Your Fraternity and Your American Heritage," arguing that the Founding Fathers "endeavored to and did establish a constitutional republic and not a democracy. A democracy would have meant rule by the majority with no protection for the rights of the minority or the individual. . . . Today there are many nice, cultured people—our friends and neighbors—and even you and I at times—who harbor the pagan belief that sacrifice of the individual serves some higher good. . . . Too many Americans believe that simple enactment of a law by the Legislature (or by the Supreme Court) makes the acts permitted legitimate without recognizing that things are not necessarily just and right because the law declares them to be so."[47] Everett made no direct comment on particular pieces of legislation and litigation, though any number of proximate examples of undue transgressions by Congress and the courts might have sprung readily to the minds of his Southern audience. Nor did he directly comment on water fluoridation. His address gracefully connected the two issues for Houston dentists without crassly mentioning either.

The insistent anticommunism of the campaign against water fluoridation built on this logic. Detroiters who opposed fluoride deployed rhetoric loaded with the psychological weight of the connection between the actions of a centralized state and the threat of Communism: the advocates of fluoride, they argued, were greedy political aggrandizers of turf, pursuing a "domino effect" that would fluoridate the growing suburban territory outside the city proper. "Since 1962, the Detroit Department of Water Supply does not recognize signs proclaiming 'City Limits.'"[48] Letters to Mayor Jerome P. Cavanaugh from local antifluoridationists were even more direct: one concluded "'Children's teeth' is only a smokescreen behind which the promters [sic] hide, the *real* purpose is to make us docile and subservient. I'm tired of socialistic schemes!"[49] Technical objections to fluoridation, on the grounds that the concentration of fluoride in public water supplies would be difficult to control, drew on the popular understanding of Communism as a stealthy threat to remind Detroiters that fluoride *"becomes more hazardous to all of us because it is colorless, odorless and tasteless."*[50] At legislative hearings about fluoride, one speaker argued that an "'iron curtain' had been dropped around Grand Rapids to hide the [negative] effects of fluoridation."[51] The notorious secrecy of the USSR was powerfully present in the minds of fluoride's opponents. One antifluoridation item in a magazine published by the Roman Catholic Scarboro Missions cited dentist J. E. Waters in *Dental Survey* claiming that "Truth will out, as even those who maintain the 'Iron Curtain' are discovering. It is to be hoped that a minimum of harm will have been done before the 'Fluorine Curtain' has been torn down and the truth given fully to the profession and the public."[52] At moments of extreme provocation, antifluoridationists argued that fluoride wasn't just metaphorically similar to Communism, but that it was actually part of a Communist plot to take over the United States. "'Dental caries' is merely a 'front' to conceal the devilish machinations of a handful of evil conspirators," wrote one in 1953. "Fluoridation has been used in countries taken over by dictators to immobilize the people's will and ability to think." Fluoride, he theorized, was being used to make port cities in the United States docile and vulnerable to Communist attack. "Inland communities that have been fluoridated are, on the whole, small towns and more easily approached by the fluoridators. This was necessary in order to avoid the appearance of attacking strategic locations only."[53]

Attitudes toward Activism

Particularly in retrospect, it is easy to mock those who opposed fluoride for their obsessiveness about Communism and their paranoia about threats to the American way of life: the unsympathetic image of General Jack D. Ripper looms large in the history of American popular culture. Other contemporaries, including many sociologists, commented more demurely on the "alienation" they imagined antifluoridationists to be experiencing. Often, they posited that sense of alienation—by which they meant a belief that one lacked effective control over one's surroundings—as the reason for the antif-luoridationists' suspicion of the motives of the government.[54]

When the moment suited them, however, antifluoridationists were as enthusiastic—and as capable—as anyone of using political activism to manipulate the mechanisms of representative democracy, suggesting that the condescending "alienation" explanation was inappropriately applied. Antif-luoridationists felt invested enough in the American political system to make able use of its tools—when fluoridation was put to a vote, it was defeated more than six times out of ten.[55] In Detroit, those who opposed fluoride mounted an aggressive campaign to defeat it in the 1965 city elections: their literature revealed that they expected representative government to function as adver-tised. "To stop the fluoridation campaign the mayor and council of Detroit and the officials of the 51 communities must have evidence that there are many people who know all the facts and don't want their drinking water medicated," one flyer argued.[56] Flyers asked citizens of Detroit and its sur-rounding suburbs to organize "friends and associates" against fluoridation, using the traditional instruments of American civic participation—the PTA, "civic, religious and business organizations," and contact with local offi-cials—to try to defeat fluoridation on the 1965 ballot. Antifluoridationists' environmental arguments against fluoride, too, were calculated to invite con-temporary clean-water and anti-pollution activists into the campaign against water fluoridation.

Faced with such an empowered opposition, dentists and others who advocated water fluoridation had to re-examine their tactics. The arguments they made, and strategies they chose, typically proceeded from their sense that dentists were experts whose judgments about measures affecting Ameri-cans' teeth ought to be trusted. Derision of people who feared negative health effects from fluoride was a popular strategy among dentists who were willing to use advanced knowledge and technical expertise as a weapon against the ill-informed rabble. In 1945, one writer reported that "An amusing example of the power of the imagination came to light when plans for placing fluorine in the water supply of one of the experimental cities were first announced. . . . A few days after the scheduled date, the city water department began to receive complaints that they were suffering from sore mouths and their teeth were changing color. City officials were sympathetic and advised the complainers to visit their dentists. Whatever was happening to their teeth had nothing to do with fluorine in the water, because no fluorine had yet been used. There had been a slight hitch in the plans, and it had been impossible to start the experiment on the date announced!"[57]

In the 1960s, this general scorn for the ill-informed was supplemented by direct ad hominem attacks on particular individuals who opposed fluoridation. At several junctures, the *Journal of the American Dental Association* published updated lists of "Comments on the Opponents of Fluoridation," which compiled the writings of antifluoridation individuals and groups in other forums for the convenient reading of ADA members. In 1965, the listing for Royal Lee, the publisher of one particularly rabid antifluoridationist's writings, included news of the Seventh Circuit Court of Appeals' upholding of his sentence for the interstate shipment of "falsely and fraudulently" labeled vitamin products. The item also cited a University of Pittsburgh dentist who said, of Lee, "I can assure you that every point made by Lee [about fluoridation] can be met with many facts, and every twist that he has given can be untwisted."[58] Partisans like Royal Lee, as the standard bearers of the antifluoridation movement, were particularly attractive targets for dentists convinced of their own professional expertise. Dentists' claim to possess elite knowledge often disgusted fluoride's opponents, who believed strongly that lay Americans were the best judges of matters affecting their own health, and rejected the idea that special expertise was necessary to produce and interpret scientific evidence, or to apply that evidence in real life. Attacks upon prominent antifluoridationists on the grounds of their lack of specialized scientific knowledge, and resultant good judgment, served to further repel those who opposed fluoride.

Fluoride's proponents, like its opponents, sought to capitalize on existing anticommunist sentiment by describing their political foes using terminology that invoked the prevailing suspicion of ideological extremism. When it worked, this strategy helped to rebut the claim that fluoride advocates were Communists themselves. During the Detroit fluoridation debates, for example, William Travis argued that opponents of fluoridation were political reactionaries who were "immune to education—totally unimpressed by scientific evidence advanced in [fluoridation's] behalf."[59] Travis also appealed to Americans' image of themselves as a modern people uniquely open to new ideas and salubrious change. Antifluoridationists, he argued, were motivated by their "dislike of change" and tendency to "always suspect the worst. Seldom has any cause rallied so many different kinds of supporters to its banner, ranging from skeptical doctors and hard-boiled citizens who just don't want their water tampered with, to a weird array of anti-Semites, charlatan diehard McCarthyites and flustered old ladies."[60]

Travis and others were particularly troubled by the highly organized nature of the anti-fluoride campaign in Detroit, where activism and political upheaval of all types were dangerously destabilizing the tense racial standoff that had prevailed in the city. They, and other dentists, were suspicious of individuals who devoted disproportionate energy to political participation. California dentist John Knutson described antifluoridationists as "professional antis"; Tennessee dentist William Wicker called them "professional 'againsters'"—with "professional," in both instances, understood as a term of derision rather than one of acclaim.[61] This characterization of antifluoridationists suggested that they had secret backing making their organizing efforts possible: "Directing the forces of the opposition are the career antifluoridationists who spread their gospel of fear of fluoridation through extensive travel and through seemingly unlimited printed matter," mused one writer in 1965.[62] This terminology resonated with the existing discourse of anticommunism, which conjured up the specter of paid agitators being deployed by the Soviets to wreck the American way of life. As a side benefit, it also invoked the image of "outside agitators" destabilizing the segregated South in this period.[63] Like Communists, antifluoridationists were described, variously, as irresponsible, deceitful, devious, frenzied, cruel, and implacable: their organizing impetus knew no ends. Many writers cautioned their audiences that antifluoridationists had been known to continue organizing opposition to fluoridation even after ballot measures had seemingly settled the question.

The effort to associate those who opposed fluoridation with ideological extremism met with limited success: the aggressive anticommunism of fluoride's opponents was just too prominent to be overlooked. As the decade wore on, dentists who experienced persistently successful arguments against fluoride as threats to the supremacy of their professional judgment began to agree that the lay public could not be relied upon to resist the pressure of antifluoridation organizers, to objectively evaluate existing scientific evidence, and to arrive at logical conclusions. "The lay public caught in the crossfire of conflicting charges," William Travis wrote in 1966, "is very often bewildered and confused. To the uninformed, both sides may sound reasonable enough, so whom is one to believe?"[64] An Oregon dentist, reflecting on a similar local controversy, made a halfhearted attempt to separate a "small but vocal minority" of antifluoridationists from the mass of the lay public who could be reached with education and political organizing. He admitted that because of the former group, organizing would need to be continuous: "The story of fluoridation's effectiveness must continue to be told no matter how impressive our victories may seem," he wrote.[65] One public health officer ventured that "If the fluoridation leaders know how people feel and what they are willing to do about what they feel, then, as the community organizers are so fond of saying, they would 'start where the people are.'"[66] But starting where the people are is time-consuming and costly, and dentists' patience with the public was waning.

Dentists' frustration with the intransigence of laypeople mirrored the discontent of other medical experts whose authority was frequently attacked by contemporary activists—feminists who argued against medical control of childbirth, for example, and black activists who portrayed medicine as the tool of a racially oppressive state.[67] The contemporary climate of increasing public skepticism about medical judgment helped persuade dentists that it was wasteful to spend prodigious amounts of time and money convincing laypeople that fluoridation was a good idea. As a result, they began to argue for removing the question of whether to fluoridate public water supplies from the hands of the public entirely, through the passage of "state-level legislation to make fluoridation mandatory in all communities."[68] In Detroit, William Travis promoted a bill removing the responsibility for decision making about fluoride from the hands of the lay public and placing it in the office of the Department of Public Health, "instead of passing the decision on to the butcher, baker, and candlestick maker!"[69] One Pennsylvania dentist wrote: "The answer is compulsory fluoridation enacted or enforced on the state level. It is inconceivable that fluoridation ever got to be considered for public debate and referenda in the first place. . . . If all the other public health measures, now commonly accepted today, were left up to each community to be settled by referenda and communal debates, a conservative estimate is that the health of the nation would be 50 years behind where we are now."[70] Advocates of fluoride agreed that decisions should be made by experts, not by members of an untrustworthy public.

Similar skepticism of lay wisdom underlay dentists' opposition to the arguments that use of fluoridated dentifrices alone could protect the American public, and that milk, instead of water, should be fluoridated on the grounds that it was easier than water for the dissenting minority to avoid. "*Who is going to fluoridate the milk??* . . ." William Travis asked. "If the housewife is expected to fluoridate the milk, then we are promoting just another *personal public health measure!!* Time and experience have adequately demonstrated that any health measure requiring any degree of inconvenience, cost, or persistent participation on the part of the individual is doomed to failure!!! I feel it is unfair, unnecessary and illogical to expect the American housewife to assume the additional chore of fluoridation of milk."[71] Travis's ire was directed in large part against the notion that fluoridation ought to be an individual choice. However, it was difficult for contemporary opponents of fluoride to separate his exasperation with this notion from his low opinion of the intelligence of the American housewife.

Dentists' belief in their professional authority, and resultant willing-ness to embrace statist authoritarianism as a means of promoting fluoride, enraged fluoride's opponents. It also chafed uncomfortably against dentists' longstanding commitment to the sanctity of individual effort and decision-making in matters of health care finance. The ADA claimed that government could not be trusted to provide health insurance no matter how badly the public wanted it, but should be trusted to fluoridate water no matter how vig-orously the public opposed it. Some dentists found the cognitive dissonance produced by these contradictory positions difficult to tolerate, and a small chorus of protest against the prevailing negative opinion of the public arose among a tiny minority of dentists who argued that the necessity of organiz-ing the community around fluoridation actually improved democracy in the United States. The public health officer who advocated meeting the people "where they are" speculated that "It could be that, through all the duress on fluoridation, we are learning something about introducing extra fiber in the processes of Democracy."[72] From Trenton, New Jersey, came the report that the capital city had been named an "All-American City" for 1965 by the National Municipal League in part because of the mobilization of more than 2,000 people "to do battle in the fluoridation war. . . . They are justifiably proud of the award which shows the way other cities and towns can become All-American."[73] In this view, it was not only fluoridation itself, but the politi-cal process of achieving it, that entitled Trenton to such a title.

Dentists and others who advocated water fluoridation longed for a world in which a health intervention that was such a self-evident scientific good would be uncontroversial. As their patience with the actual political climate with which they had to contend wore thin, humor emerged: in 1968, reporters for the *Dental Students' Magazine* reported on their "pilgrimage" to Newburgh, New York, highlighting the acceptance of fluoridation there by recounting their attempts to find "plaques or markers in town commemorating fluorida-tion." "We asked the pretty desk clerk at the motel if there were any. . . . She was genuinely puzzled. 'Flora Who?' . . . So we asked the maid—a beaming, motherly type—if she knew that fluoridation occurred here as early as 1946. Immediately her demeanor changed. 'I don't know anything about anybody's defloration,' she said with finality."[74] Another tack sought to minimize the question by inserting the drama of fluoride refusal into a cliché domestic scenario: a 1965 cartoon in the *Journal of the American Dental Association* depicted a businessman, just home from work and reading the evening paper, gruffly telling his hovering wife "I will NOT drink a fluoridated martini."[75]

These attempts at minimization through humor fell short, however, because the subject they sought to trivialize was so inextricably bound up with contested ideas about science, aesthetics, and politics. Would fluoride harm Americans' teeth or help them? What counted as help—and what as harm? Who could demand help—and from whom? Who should decide? These questions, vigorously debated but never resolved, would re-emerge in other debates about dental care and the state of the dental profession near the end of the twentieth century.

The relative success of campaigns for the fluoridation of public water supplies marked the apex of dentists' drive for professional legitimacy as guardians of public health. Their influence over an important public health policy meant that their battle for status equal with that of physicians was closer than it had ever been to fruition. To achieve that success, dentists had been forced to cooperate with state authority in a way that made them uncomfortable. The vehement anti-statist analysis articulated by antifluoridationists hewed close to the positions dentists had traditionally taken about state interventions in dental care—and particularly dental care financing. Dentists' frustrating encounters with the rough-and-tumble of electoral political battles over fluoride offended their belief that scientific expertise and training ought to be the tickets to participation in scientific debates, souring them further on the wisdom of a centralized governmental power that could so easily be manipulated by populist demagogues. Together with dentists' anger over increasing governmental incursions into their entrepreneurial opportunities, the fluoride debates set the stage for a backlash against public health dentistry, and dramatically increased interest in individual aesthetic interventions, both within and outside the profession.

Chapter 6

The "Satisfaction of Dentistry" and the End of Public Health

Fluoride left dentists facing the prospect of markedly reduced income from restorative work. Studies showed that the reduction of tooth decay not only led to fewer fillings and extractions but, with less room for teeth to move about haphazardly in Americans' mouths, to lower rates of malocclusion, suggesting that Americans' need for orthodontic services might also drop in fluoride's wake.[1] Some dentists were optimistic that a lowered need for reparative care might mean that they would have more time to engage in planned preventative treatment. More powerful figures perceived the possibility of a lowered volume of business as a serious threat. It was, they felt, of a piece with other, more pernicious changes marking the efforts of non-dentists to get something for nothing—and usually at dentists' expense.

In the decades that followed the widespread fluoridation of public water supplies, these dentists found themselves retrenching against a barrage of internal and external challenges to the viability of "American dentistry" as a profession of high social, economic, and scientific standing. The relationship between these challenges and the idea of collective action for the public good further encouraged American dentists to see the notion of collective public engagement itself as a threat, rather than an opportunity. Social movements questioning or rejecting existing race and gender relationships plagued dentists, and the license for unfettered action they believed they had won for their profession. Their female assistants, long conceived as subservient helpmeets, started to seem like potential or actual advocates of feminist liberation on the job—or, still worse, as organizers of unions. The historical white dominance of the dental profession was challenged by black dentists' efforts to achieve fully equal treatment within the ADA. Black dentists, through their own national organization, opposed the ADA's resistance to programs like Medicare and Social Security. To the leaders and active members of the ADA, this portended the ways in which the policy positions of a fully integrated ADA might have to change, softening toward undesirable "big government" social programs in order to reflect the opinions of an integrated membership.

Most importantly, renewed proposals for publicly provided health insurance seemed to use the notion of shared risk and responsibility in ways that would impinge on dentists' professional prerogatives and success. The lived reality of even voluntary insurance, dentists felt, was already proving damaging. By the early 1960s, over one million Americans were enrolled in dental insurance plans;[2] nearly one-third of all American medical expenditures were paid for through insurance.[3] Increasingly aggressive legislative efforts to ensure government provision of health care to the needy struck fear in the hearts of dentists. The advent of Medicare and Medicaid, resisted by—but thrust upon—their physician counterparts, gave them grave concerns about the future of their income streams and their standing as autonomous entrepreneurs. Like physicians, they vigorously opposed the prospect of systematic change that threatened the basic economic organization of their profession.

Dentists' renewed insistence on the primacy of private practice was of a piece with more widely embraced changes in the concept of American citizenship, which was increasingly linked in the postwar period with status as a consumer of both private enterprise and government.[4] Arguments for patients' self-reliance, and against the expansion of free or subsidized dental care, sprang from dentists' genuinely held sensibilities about the proper scope of government and the role of the private citizen, increasingly represented by the New Right's opposition to New Deal expansion of government involvement in Americans' lives. Such arguments also reflected more cynical interests in preserving the race, gender, and entrepreneurial prerogatives of mostly white, and overwhelmingly male, dentists.

At the end of the twentieth century, the dentists represented by the American Dental Association quietly withdrew their support of most non-fluoride public health programs, and articulated a reconfigured discourse of Americanism in dentistry. In this new ideological schema, the fact that even a socially and professionally conservative organization like the ADA had once considered Americans' dental health a proper subject for community concern and intervention would have no place. Dentists shuttered school and industrial dental hygiene programs, as they had closed most public dental dispensaries decades before. They had delivered to Americans the great gift of fluoride. By the middle of the 1960s, threats to their income and professional prerogatives seemed like a snub to the profession's earlier largesse. As one ADA film for dentists observed: "Mindblower . . . Dentists Under Siege."[5]

The Rebellion of the Office Wife

Among the trends that distressed dentists was their sense that they were losing the control they had once enjoyed over their offices—and particularly over their office personnel. Increasingly, the technical, business, and demographic demands of the postwar period required that dentists employ assistants and hygienists to work in their offices. There were new office machines to be operated, and an ever-diversifying range of supplies and equipment to be selected, ordered, and maintained: dentists considered these tasks both bewildering and degrading. The surge in the population of youth caused by the postwar baby boom also seemed to call for more paraprofessional assistance from dental hygienists and assistants, who were reputed to be particularly effective managers of children. At times, these auxiliaries took their place by the sides of women receptionists or billing clerks, who were already familiar faces in the dental suite. In 1960, one Akron dentist reported that a study of dental practices had yielded the news that 88 percent of dentists employed "auxiliary help," in numbers ranging from one person (in 44 percent of offices) to five (in 3 percent).[6] These "auxiliary helpers" provided an enormous competitive advantage to their employers, increasing the net income of their offices on an almost one-to-one basis (such that "the dentist with four and a half assistants has a net income almost four times greater than the dentist who works alone"[7]). Very few dentists quibbled with the proposition that having a woman employed as an assistant or a hygienist was important to effective practice management.

Dentists had long considered women—particularly good-looking women—to be the ideal candidates for dental assistant and dental hygienist positions. In the late twentieth century, dentists' construction of auxiliary dental personnel as comely customer service providers, combined with the currency of the gender analysis proffered by second-wave feminism, resulted in new tensions on the job. Dental assistants and hygienists were expected to emphasize their pulchritude at work. A 1967 article discussing the characteristics of the "ideal D.A." listed "Attractiveness" and "Femininity" as the first and second most important qualities, before "Efficiency," "Brains," or

"Education," which were listed fourth, sixth, and last.[8] One writer encouraged women assistants to contemplate the sorry case of "Carlotta," who arrived late to work one day "muttering apologies and breathlessly explaining that the doctor would be along in a moment. . . . [The] patient looked at her again and shook his head firmly. 'This is not the type of girl,' he said to himself, 'that I would choose to put her finger in *my* mouth.'" The author, a dentist, mused: "Since this is one criterion whereby nearly all adult male patients judge the delectableness of a dental assistant, let us discuss how a conflict of images has caused Carlotta to be rejected so decisively."[9] Some dentists congratulated one another for having managed to hire particularly attractive office personnel: writing to dentists of his experience at the annual New Orleans Dental Conference, George Crane said that he had "long noted the good eyesight of you dental surgeons when it comes to picking wives, dental assistants, and dental hygienists."[10]

The elision of the boundaries between office staff and spouses created friction in the workplace. Consistently sexualized on the job, women employed by dentists found themselves the objects of concern from dentists' wives, who were offered columns of their own explaining how to deal with "The Other Women in Your Husband's Life!"[11] Even as they were being jealously watched as threats to dentists' marriages, they were expected to use their feminine dignity to throw a cloak of purity around otherwise prurient-seeming situations, as when a woman was placed under anesthesia by a lone male dentist. However, the knotty problem of delicate women assistants' vulnerability to the sexual advances of male patients was typically ignored.[12] To the contrary, some sources seemed to suggest that the presence of women in the office could be sexually unsettling to male patients: one cartoon, for example, showed a timid-looking man in a dental chair with his head cradled between the breasts of a stoic-looking assistant. Gesticulating toward a broken headrest, the dentist said "I'm sorry, Mr. Crumbly, our head rest won't be repaired until next week."[13] No dental journal, and no publication for dental assistants, ever addressed what assistants ought to do if they were being harassed by their male employers.

Despite this hodgepodge of mutually contradictory perceptions of women's sexual power—or perhaps because of it—they were regularly enjoined to avoid asserting themselves as non-sexual professionals at work. Women dental employees who did so could expect to be the targets of derision for their overdeveloped senses of self-importance. In one cartoon in *CAL*, a magazine produced by the Coe Alginate Laboratories dental supply company for dental assistants, for example, women in nursing attire stood by the door of a dental office, which was marked "J. W. Grom, DDS" in small type and "Miss Jones, CDA." in a much larger font. "I understand she's a rather forceful dental assistant," one woman observer said to the other. Encouraged to avoid directness, dental assistants in the late twentieth century agonized over how to raise matters such as salary and vacation time. One who identified herself as "Fran" complained to an advice column for dental assistants that her employer, who was also part owner of a beauty shop, paid her only sixty dollars a week and the beauticians ninety dollars a week—because, he said, "Those beauticians have to work so hard!"[14] Fran asked the readers of the "Problem of the Month" column to send her advice through the journal: "If my doctor ever learned I wrote to *CAL* I'd die," she wrote.[15] The first-prize advice published four months later (whose author received ten dollars) admonished Fran to consider her own culpability in her low pay: because women often expected to quit work after marriage, "we may not always prepare for our profession as carefully as we should," she wrote. She advised Fran to have "a heart-to-heart" talk with her employer, and then to consider quitting her job.[16] The second-prize winner advised Fran to discuss her salary with her employer in a straightforward and direct manner, keeping in mind that "an employee has only to accept or reject," not to negotiate.[17] Not all dental assistants were as conciliatory as those whose advice was published in *CAL*: the intransigent opinions of experienced dental assistants, and their propensity for expressing those opinions directly, caused dentists throughout the twentieth century to advise hiring completely inexperienced assistants whenever possible.[18]

Dentists attempted to keep women employees dependent upon them for compensation and information. But the increasingly visible challenges posed by feminism, the advent of the sex-discrimination protections in the 1964 Civil Rights Act, and the boom in the unionization for collective bargaining of women employees in traditionally female occupations like teaching, nursing and secretarial work in the 1960s and 1970s had major impacts on women's expectations about how they would be treated on the job.[19] Dentists feared the prospect of losing control over employees who felt justified in demanding more equitable treatment. They objected to the federal government's attempts to force the issue of gender equity at work: contemplating the "shock" that might afflict someone who found him or herself being treated by a male dental assistant, one dental journal editor mused that "it would have been better if Congress had just abolished sex itself"—a prospect which, by its very impossibility, seemed to highlight the ludicrousness of legislative

attempts to ensure equity in hiring and treatment by employers.[20] Dentists
lodged equally strong objections to the prospect of their employees organizing into unions: in 1965, for example, a lawyer from the union-busting Los
Angeles firm Iverson and Hogoboom was brought in to present to the Southern California State Dental Association on "what you as employers can do to
combat unionism within the letter and spirit of public policy."[21] Dental office
employees rarely attempted to organize, but the prospect that they would do
so scared dentists enough to prompt changes in their behavior as managers. One California dentist promoted generous employee benefit plans for
hygienists and assistants as a means of "excluding union interference." The
article in which he outlined his plan featured a sketch, in ominous marker
strokes, of a dental nurse in white, looming over the viewer while carrying a
picket sign that read "unfair."[22]

Together with new federal attention to workplace equity issues, the
threat of union organizing by dental auxiliaries changed the employment
practices of dental offices. Slowly, articles counseling dentists to avoid hiring women who wore too much makeup, or whose uniforms showed "panty
lines," were replaced by descriptions of the most legally unimpeachable
ways of conducting annual salary reviews of dental hygienists. When labor
strife in the dental office persisted, employees had a new way to redress their
grievances: in 1977, "Anonymous" reported to *Dental Economics*, in much
the style of the tabloid women's magazines, that "A Disgruntled Employee
Took Me to Labor Court."[23]

Political Activity by African American Dentists

Like women dental auxiliaries, black dentists of the late twentieth century
organized to bring more equity to the dental workplace, making the longstanding racial segregation of the dental profession less and less tenable.
The racial discrimination in the application of the GI bill that occurred
in the wake of World War II heightened the disparity of views and experiences that perennially attended the racial divide in the profession. During the 1950s, the journal of the National Dental Association periodically
reported on the policies of the state and local dental societies that constituted the ADA: in 1954, for example, the Kansas City District Dental Society
rejected the applications of six black NDA members for local membership.
(The white president of the society, asked to comment, reportedly said that
the vote "speaks for itself," a comment which was apparently intended to
communicate endorsement of the prevailing policy of racial segregation.[24])

In the same year, an item titled "Great Expectations?" heralded the Georgia Dental Association's decision to invite "the Negro dentists of Georgia" to attend scientific sessions of the annual meeting—though not to be admitted to membership. "Twenty-five of these dentists did attend the meeting," the journal reported, "with benefit to themselves and without incident or interference with anyone else in attendance."[25] Black dental leaders were careful to admonish readers to do their part for integration by being well prepared for the meetings and conferences they attended. "It seems appropriate in the light of these happenings to reemphasize the fact that it is absolutely essential for those dentists belonging to minority groups to be prepared and familiar with current scientific thought, with organizational methods, with professional trends and with inter-professional policies."[26]

In the 1960s, black dentists who had been firm but cautious advocates for integration greeted the promises of the Great Society and the civil rights movement with enthusiasm. Their activism in these matters received a lukewarm reception among whites. Like the American Medical Association, the predominantly white ADA called upon the "American" values of individualism and entrepreneurship in opposition to Medicare, Medicaid, affirmative action in dental school admission, and federal aid for dental school education. In contrast, the predominantly black National Dental Association cited the American ideals of inclusiveness and equality in its support of the very same programs.[27] For example, white dentists in Texas in 1962 were treated to the reprinting of a pamphlet titled "Social Security: Facts and Fantasy" by their state dental association, including the dire prediction that "Most persons in the lower income brackets will by 1970 be paying higher taxes for Social Security than for income."[28] Black dentists who read the *Bulletin of the National Dental Association* in 1958 were informed, in optimistic contrast, that Social Security "provides a basis or foundation upon which one can build toward freedom of worry."[29]

Black dentists had always conceived of the scope of their professional responsibilities broadly. In their minds, the professional skills of those who had to struggle so mightily for education and professional acceptance should be used not only to diagnose dental disease, but to identify social sickness and to advance the status of black Americans as a group. When the *Quarterly*'s editor, prominent black dentist Clifton Dummett, memorialized Martin Luther King Jr. in July of 1968, he argued that "As a member of the health professions it seems to me that his message and legacy are crystal clear. With acute perception and without rancor, he diagnosed the all-pervading sickness gnawing at the very vitality of this land he loved deeply."[30] The journal clearly conceived of itself as an organ of racial uplift as well as of professional correspondence, and often published political items of interest to black professionals, including, at times, the addresses of major black American political figures to the association's meetings. In 1970, civil rights activist Julian Bond addressed the NDA, urging that "The day must come when government ensures that every person has guaranteed medical and dental care, and that every person in need has a hospital bed."[31] The *Quarterly* reprinted this section of Bond's speech, describing Bond favorably as "the dynamic, young Georgian," and offering its readers the opportunity to identify with Bond's position as that of the association itself.[32] In 1972, similarly, Michigan congressman John Conyers appeared before the association to map out "Black Political Strategy for 1972," calling on black professionals to "unify the black community and to develop a strategy to effect a permanent cure for a sick nation."[33]

The "sick nation" rhetoric of the civil rights and black power movements helped to mark the divide between the law-abiding, God-fearing Americans who voted for Richard Nixon and the young idealists who populated the social-justice movements of the era. In their aspirations to middle-class status, black dentists straddled the gap between the two groups, sometimes awkwardly. In the 1960s and 1970s, the journal of the NDA was tightly controlled by Clifton Dummett, who articulated a philosophy of professional engagement that hybridized Booker T. Washington's vision of racial self-reliance with W.E.B. Du Bois's plan for racial integration as achieved by a "talented tenth." Dummett believed that each individual black practitioner of dentistry was responsible for the success or failure of the whole body. He demanded strict personal discipline from individual dentists in the service of the profession, the race, and the nation, whose interests he saw as congruent. In October 1971, for example, a testy Dummett dressed down the journal's readers, pointing out that press coverage of that year's annual convention featured them discussing the potential financial gain to be had from taking on welfare patients, and not reflecting on how to "help people to help themselves. . . . The responsibility for this adverse publicity must be borne by those black dentists whose remarks provided the basis for the news stories."[34] He considered it important that the NDA stand for a particular kind of citizenship—one of group struggle toward success.

Black professionals of all sorts, but particularly in health care, shared Dummett's sense of individual responsibility for the fate of the larger group.[35] The social expectations that prevailed as a result could prove particularly

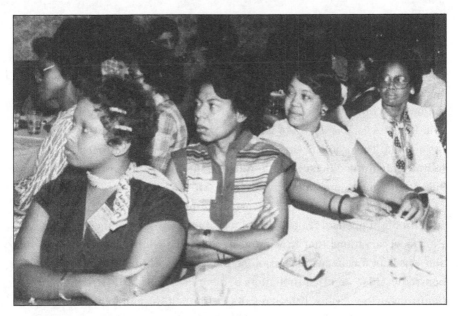

Figure 8 Dental hygienists looked unhappy with the content of a lecture on "sexology" at a meeting of the National Dental Association, 1977. *Quarterly of the National Dental Association* 36 (October 1977): 25.

stifling to professional black women, who were expected to achieve a racially transgressive level of success while abiding by middle-class gender norms. Though the NDA's journal promoted the advancement of black women in dentistry, published items, particularly about professional conferences that brought together black dentists and dental hygienists, consistently sexualized and patronized women. In 1977, the photo layout of four black women dental hygienists at the annual NDA conference was subtitled: "The Dental Hygienists went to school. They took a course in sexology and paid serious attention to the speaker who told them to 'assert yourself.'"[36] In the following year, a photo of two young black women in evening wear was titled: "Bubbling Brown Sugar! We're glad you came!"[37]

When the imperatives of racial equality and gender equity clashed in the NDA journal, it mirrored the "double bind" that black women experienced elsewhere in American culture, and particularly the version of that bind that prevailed on middle-class black women. Elsewhere in the black media, professional black women were often positioned as the arbiters of a higher, more "scientific" standard of living for black Americans in general. The bourgeois black magazine *Ebony*, for instance, periodically profiled black medical and dental practitioners, repeatedly mentioning their frustration with black Americans' poor understanding of the principles of good health. One feature article on dentist Linda Smith announced: "She tries to raise 'dental IQ' in Black people."[38] In return for the respect they were accorded as professionals, women like Linda Smith were expected to demonstrate proper respect for the middle-class gender values to which *Ebony* editors imagined that their readers aspired. The profile of Dr. Smith was careful to point out that she spent her (admittedly limited) leisure time "relaxing quietly with a young doctor whom she dates," and commented approvingly on the tasteful décor of her apartment.[39] A similar profile of Northwestern University School of Dentistry dean Juliann Bluitt opened: "She doesn't look like a dentist,"[40] and concluded with Bluitt's observations that "a woman has a responsibility in the home," that she was "not a women's liberationist, believe me, although my life seems to contradict this," and that in matters of dental school administration, "a bit of 'feminine maneuvering' brings results."[41] Implicit in such items was the message that professional success could be received as a positive good, as long as the women who achieved it were sure to pay due respect to gender norms.

Black and white male dentists struggled to make sense of the increasing presence of women in professional life, but the intractable differences between the two groups on the subjects of racial integration and politics far outweighed the similarity of their experiences around gender. These differences were rarely reflected in direct public dispute about dental topics: the ADA and its constituent societies had more money and greater access to the media than did the NDA, and the NDA could hardly hope to mount a successful opposition to such a powerful organization on matters of policy. The differences between the two groups were, however, played out in challenges to the discriminatory practices of the ADA in the 1950s, 1960s, and 1970s. Individual black dentists began questioning, and then litigating, the ADA-affiliated state societies' policies of racial exclusion.[42] The pages of major national dental journals—both black and white—reflected the tension that resulted.

In June of 1964, for example, the *Journal of the American Dental Association* published a filler item, titled "The Color Guard," disparaging a dentist "in one of the nation's large cities, who refused emergency treatment to a young Negro woman."[43] This was a comparatively bold move on the part of *JADA*'s editors, who had also quietly begun to insert photographs featuring black members—and joint meetings of ADA and NDA leaders—in the journal. In response to the letter about the dentist who had refused to treat the young black woman, one Ohio reader wrote to concur that "the incident described in your editorial is not uncommon; rather it occurs frequently and in most communities at one time or another."[44] But James Webb of Lamarque, Texas, returned his copy of the June volume of *JADA* to the editorial office, writing: "As I began to read the Reports of Councils and Bureaus and the News of Dentistry Sections, I was confronted with a succession of pictures of our officers and fellow dentists eating, visiting, awarding, and in general making up to Negroes of various minor positions. Then, to cap it off, I was hit with an editorial trying to tell me whom I can and cannot treat in my office. I believe this organization is supposed to represent the feelings of the majority of dentists in this country, and I can't believe we are all in accordance with the kind of stuff you are printing. When the ADA publication returns to being a professional journal instead of a monthly newsletter for the NAACP, start sending it again."[45]

Webb's letter touched off a firestorm of comment that persisted into the October issue of the journal. Another Texas reader wrote, sympathetically, that dentists who felt they could not render their best service, for any reason including their own intolerance, were entitled to turn away patients.[46] Others replied that they regretted seeing the two Texans' letters in the *Journal* at all, and that the sentiments expressed therein highlighted the need for the profession to develop an enforceable code of ethics that would forbid racial discrimination by dentists. Some state and local societies were, at the same time, actively defending their rights to discriminate. In 1964, for example, North Carolina dentist Reginald Hawkins, who was the chairman of the civil rights committee of the NDA, sued the North Carolina Dental Society (a constituent of the ADA), which had refused him membership because he was black. Hawkins argued that the dental society, because it effectively appointed the members of the state's Board of Dental Examiners, was an agency of the state, and therefore subject to the provisions of the Fourteenth Amendment.[47] Rejecting tolerance for slow change, Hawkins described the ADA as "aloof. . . . They've allowed these eleven states [which excluded black dentists from membership] to send delegates and help make ADA policy for all other states, knowing full well that Negroes were not adequately represented. Oh, yes, the ADA has made pronouncements. But there's a difference between pronouncements and action."[48]

The racial politics of the ADA liberalized over time, particularly after the assassination of John F. Kennedy. That change in mores, together with Hawkins's lawsuit and other similar legal challenges, prompted the ADA's

House of Delegates to forward to the 1965 annual convention the identical proposals advanced by the Michigan and New York state dental societies "requesting the elimination of discrimination against Negro dentists who apply for membership in organized dentistry."[49] Sentiment about the integration of the profession was by no means unified. The editors of *JADA* hoped to take a position that would alienate as few dentists as possible. In an attempt to pacify integrationists, they endorsed the proposal. They made a conciliatory gesture toward segregationists who blamed blacks for their own social isolation from whites, counseling that, should the proposal pass, "nonmember dentists who reside in states, including those in the North, where discriminatory practices do not exist . . . [should] exhibit their sincerity by becoming active members of organized dentistry."[50] The proposals passed, and the following year, the president of the ADA appeared at a banquet dinner at the NDA's annual meeting to "bring cordial greetings from the American Dental Association, its officers and trustees," and to invite NDA members who visited Chicago to "plan a tour of the magnificent new home of the ADA . . . I am certain it will impress you with its functional design and architectural splendor."[51]

Despite such overtures by the ADA, black dentists clearly did not trust that their political positions would be fairly represented in the integrated organization. In 1967, when the dean of the Howard University College of Dentistry proposed that the NDA "cease to exist as we know it today" on the grounds that the ADA had finally been integrated, he suggested not that the organization dissolve but that it give up its "scientific" functions and "continue to exist . . . as a strong social and political action force in the mainstream."[52] The minority of black dentists who were "financial members"[53] of the NDA, and who were the implied audience of its publications, either did not support, or were not understood by NDA leaders as supporting, the turn toward political and economic conservatism under way in the ADA during the same period. The NDA sustained a strong organizational interest in addressing the health effects of poverty and racism; in the second half of the twentieth century, the ADA rarely entertained such questions.

The Involvement of Government and
Insurance Companies in Dental Care

Like the struggle for the fluoridation of public water supplies, second-wave feminism and the encroaching demands of the civil rights movement gave the dentists represented by the ADA reason to question the logic of collective action. It was the growth of public- and private-sector programs for third-party payment of dental care that sealed their distaste for community-level solutions to individual problems. Such programs struck at dentists' short- and long-term financial interests, and at their cherished image of themselves as independent entrepreneurs. They feared and opposed the restraints on dental practice that they believed would come with dental insurance, and with increasing government involvement in providing it.

Though medical and dental opposition to national health insurance had halted a broad socialization of health and dental care costs in the post-war period, American workers in the 1950s and 1960s continued to demand health and dental benefits from their employers. Some experts believed that, by 1970, half of all of the dental care provided in the United States would be paid for through dental insurance plans.[54] The employee-benefits providers' first efforts in the direction of dental insurance consisted of what dentists referred to, disparagingly, as "closed-panel" dentistry: certain providers "participated" in the insurance plan, and employees could visit those providers, but not others, for their dental care. Dentists objected to these plans because unions and employers, not dentists, determined which providers were qualified to participate in any given plan, thereby eroding the professional autonomy of dentists. Joseph Bloom, a New Jersey dentist who authored an exposé of a local dental insurance plan titled "I Resigned from the Group Health Dental Insurance Program," complained that he had experienced a great deal of difficulty convincing the insurance company's underwriters to make appropriate allowances for complicated surgeries. "However," he noted, "when the problems were presented to the responsible officers of the union, the entire matter was corrected to the satisfaction of dentistry within a short time. It is an unfortunate truth that to correct this inequity, organized dentistry had no power to influence reasonable demands on underwriters and management, but when faced with the threat of a strike to enforce the same demands from unions, they acquiesced."[55] The fact that labor power worked more effectively than professional authority to sway third-party payers rankled Bloom. When the naked pecuniary self-interest of labor unions received more consideration than the objective professional judgment of a licensed dentist, things were in a sorry state indeed.

In an attempt to short-circuit the demand for "closed-panel" systems, state dental associations spent much of the early 1960s designing "dental service corporations"—prepaid service plans, modeled on Blue Cross and Blue Shield, whose provider pools mirrored the membership of the state association.

Proponents argued that because dental insurance of some sort was a foregone conclusion, dentists should work to be certain they would control the terms on which it was offered. Yet even these moderate movements away from fee-for-service practice angered some dentists who were members of the state dental associations. They assailed the "political leadership" of the state and national organizations for abandoning their commitments to American dental entrepreneurship. For example, a Californian blamed the ADA and its con-stituent state societies for having failed to articulate arguments against ser-vice corporations: "The powerful union trusts demanding a dental care plan," he wrote, "were like bringing up the artillery, and the barrage staggered the officers of the day who immediately retrenched into their cloister and nepo-tism and autocracy."[56] One Texas dentist wrote: "I am opposed to the Dental Service Corporation for many reasons, but primarily because it marks a devia-tion away from the private enterprise system of health service which has been responsible for developing the highest level of dentistry the world has ever known toward a form of socialized health service. . . . Service Corporations, like governments, can become hydra-headed monsters enslaving the dentist rather than serving him."[57] In response to his state dental association's move-ments to form a service corporation, one California dentist proclaimed: "I love to be my own boss. I love the free enterprise system. I love Americanism. I paid the price in full to be my own boss. I don't want to work for a corporation. . . . I do not believe the general membership of the American Dental Association who are aware of the truth will want to support this organization."[58]

Dentists' concerns about insurance reflected their ideological interest in entrepreneurial independence and their more mundane pecuniary interest in financial success. Those concerns also reflected their genuine preferences for retaining control over their day-to-day work lives and over the terms of their relationships with patients. In the 1960s, they expressed contempt for a variety of modern measures that put distance between patients and health care providers—not just those that carried a direct potential for impact on their own incomes. The modern hospital, some speculated, could force an unnatural schism between the dentist and his patient just as effectively as the health insurance company could. In 1963, one writer chided dentists to avoid practicing in hospital settings, cautioning that "dental surgeons are the last bulwark of private medical practice, for the dental surgeon still teaches his patients to come to a private office located in some downtown building or suburban office suite [instead of to a hospital, which] 'presages a shift in public allegiance to 'buildings' instead of 'men,' which precedes socialized medicine. . . . continue to make your patients obey your dictates and come to your private office!'" [59] Other contemporary conveniences, in this view, could be every bit as dangerous: in 1968, the new journal *Dental Management* published an article on the "Cause and Cure of the Cash Register Complex," arguing that the sacred dentist-patient relationship was being eroded by such pernicious modern inventions as the clipboard (which smacked of the "employment office"), the appointment-confirmation telephone call (which "eliminates the patient's responsibility for his own care"), and high reception room counters sized for the convenience of patients who wrote checks for dental service while standing—the author argued that it would be much more courteous, and therefore more reflective of the traditional dentist-patient relationship, for the patient to be invited to sit.[60] The author of "Cause and Cure of the Cash Register Complex" explicitly connected her advice about practice management with the rhetoric about contemporary battles over insurance: "It's time that everyone in the profession recognized the dehumanization process now going on," she proclaimed, "and made a full effort to keep dental care on a people-to-people basis."[61] Try as they might to turn back the tide, however, dentists in the 1960s and 1970s found themselves facing a colder, more impersonal world on all fronts. Patients increasingly regarded their services as necessary evils which were to be paid for out of pocket only in cases of extreme necessity. Meanwhile, insurance companies and government demanded accountings of professional services that dentists had once delivered, and of prices that they had once set, without interference.

One of the reasons dentists in the 1960s and 1970s found these trends so disturbing was because they were under the mistaken impression that increasing patients' access to dental care by reducing their out-of-pocket costs was a new idea. In the years after the widespread fluoridation of public water supplies, school dental hygiene programs ground to a halt: alarmed by threats to their incomes and professional autonomy, dentists erased from the shared memory of the profession the history of public health promotional campaigns, led by luminaries of the field, which had cooperated with schools and city governments to give away dental care for free. Many writers who tried to sketch out the history of dentistry—and particularly the history of dental public health—erroneously argued that government interest in providing for Americans' dental health was a new phenomenon. "It is only since the mid-1960s that the growth of government supported dental programs and the advent of proposals for national health insurance that there has been an increased awareness by private practitioners of the activities of public health dentists [sic]," one professor of dental public health proclaimed.[62] The winning entry in one dental-student essay contest argued that "traditionally, the role of dentistry has been to provide a service to the individual through a private and personal interaction between doctor and patient. . . . The practitioner . . . based his practice on the premise that 'the responsibility for the health of the American people is first of the individual, the community, the state, and the nation, in that order.'"[63]

Dentists' positive attitude toward individual entrepreneurial spirit was consistent with their earlier advocacy against "big government" solutions to Americans' health care needs. In the late twentieth century, new hostility toward collective engagement animated dentists' opposition to health and dental insurance. "From infancy," the president of the Great Lakes Society of Orthodontists wrote, "this has been a vigorous nation—made strong by millions of people who have made every possible effort to gain the rewards of self-reliant living. It is apparent on all sides that our inner strength has started to ebb. A sickness threatens to drain the character of the American people. It has been stated that this is our real health problem. We are letting a sorry wish for care-by-government deaden the urge for self-care."[64] It was almost as though the publicly funded dental hygiene programs of the 1910s, 1920s and 1930s—and the even more recent fight for the fluoridation of public water supplies in the 1950s and 1960s—had never existed. In the surging economic environment of the postwar years, dentists felt that they could count on sufficient income from private-pay patients; there no longer seemed to be any financial reason to strike the balance between "free enterprise" and free access to health care on the patients' side. The idea that it had ever been otherwise seemed, if not a nightmare, then a distantly receding dream.

Unfortunately for dentists, the "sorry wish for care-by-government" was contagious. As witnessed in part by their insistence on government- or employer-provided health care, patients were feeling less and less inclined to pay out of pocket for any kind of health care, dentistry included. "There is a growing belief," one dental student wrote, "that everyone who needs it is entitled to at least minimal dental care."[65] Patients' sense that the government had a special obligation to provide them with health and dental care (or at least health and dental insurance) seemed coupled with a dangerous demystification of dentistry's importance. Dentists complained that patients put dental care on a par with other commercial goods, rather than giving it the pride of place—and budget—to which it was entitled. "On entering dental school, I was instilled with the idea that dentistry was a health service and not a commodity to be 'sold' like refrigerators," one dentist griped. "Is it below the dignity and ethics of the profession to place dental services in the category of commercial products? I think so."[66] Some writers who commented on practice management issues argued that dentists' insistence on attending to the business side of dental care—by demanding that patients fill out multiple forms or submit to credit checks, or by adopting the structural implements of the modern business office—had incorrectly given patients the sense that the dental office was primarily a place of business rather than a site for the provision of health care, a place of industry rather than craft. "This is not a business office where the receptionist screens out overbearing salesmen," one writer complained, "This is a dentist's office. . . . In no way should it look like, function like, or be like a business office."[67] Others believed that the deep recession of the early 1970s was having an impact on patients' appraisal of all purchasing decisions—and that health care, particularly in such a feeble economic environment, simply moved from being a "need" to being an optional "want" for most patients.

Whatever the reason for patients' intransigence, dentists were faced with a quandary. Forces from within and without threatened the control they had managed to achieve over their professional lives. The social movements of the 1960s and early 1970s altered social norms around such contentious issues as gender and race, and challenged the status quo within dentistry. Those movements reflected a broader resurgence of Americans' sympathy for systematic solutions to problems that dentists had increasing motive to regard as individual concerns. But opposition to social change sparked countermovements that gave dentists the language with which to resist dramatic alteration in the economics of their profession.

Insurance, whether privately provided or sponsored by the government, endangered dentists' incomes and their control over dentistry. Nearing the end of the century, dentists who hoped to stave off insurance programs—whether public or private—confronted an array of pressing questions. How could patients be convinced to value dental care more highly? What might make them more willing to seek and pay out of pocket for expensive dental services? How could patients be "reminded"—if they had ever really known it to begin with—that dental care was the responsibility of the individual first, and the state last? And what dental interventions could help to "sell" a vision of Americanism in which the individual, rather than the group, bore the burden for his own dental health—indeed, for almost all of his needs and desires?

Chapter 7

The Look of the American Mouth

As dentists groped for measures that would restore dentistry's status and the financial potential of dentistry as a business, catering to late-twentieth-century Americans' ever-heightening interest in personal appearance seemed like a wise business decision. For these practitioners, offering high-end prosthetic services, tooth whitening procedures, and especially orthodontic care appeared an obvious choice. While the technological and cultural underpinnings of orthodontics existed early in the twentieth century, the sheer volume of reparative dental service that was necessary in the years before fluoride made orthodontic care, and the aggressive manipulation of already-available ideas about beauty and success, a low priority for both dentists and patients. Just as important as the effects of fluoridation, however, were the other reasons why orthodontics was marketed more enthusiastically, and embraced with more fervor, after the middle of the century. Until the middle of the 1950s, dentists hoped that they could demonstrate the value of their expertise through more broadly-ranging public health interventions. Political and cultural conditions unique to the end of the century, and dentists' renewed fears for their income stability, militated in the direction of stepping up the sale of orthodontics.

The postwar population boom resulted in an unusually large number of children of prime orthodontic age: their youth made them more susceptible both to orthodontic care and to the gospel of a lifetime of dentistry, inculcated in the orthodontist's chair. Surveying the demographic shift, many commentators even foresaw a time when a future glut of adult patients might make a mockery of dentists' fears about reduced demand for dental care. They argued that because of the pressure that the baby boom would put on "traditional" fee-for-service dentistry, providing comprehensive care for children and reducing the need for dental care in adults of the future was the only way to protect dentists' entrepreneurial prerogatives and incomes in both the short and the long term.[1]

Though dentists disdained insurance, some dental insurance plans covered, or partially covered, orthodontic care. Despite dentists' fears about the possibility that patients would undervalue care for which they did not pay, insurance coverage served to normalize orthodontic care, stimulating patient and parent interest in it. Reflecting the financial interests of insurers, however, almost no dental plan covered the entire cost. The practice of orthodontics was thus one of the few specialties in which dentists could anticipate having, at least for some portion of treatment, a "traditional" fee-for-service relationship with their patients. Dentists highly prized the private payment of dental bills because they believed that it would help patients to understand the true value of dentists' services. Orthodontics exceeded even the benefits of private payment itself in this regard, requiring protracted attention and participation on the part of the patient—and, often, his or her parents. There was virtually no specialty better designed to impress upon the patient that he was primarily responsible for his or her own dental health.

Orthodontics also had the distinct advantage of drawing on a long American history of linkage between appearance and individual sense of self-worth, which reached fruition in the personal-improvement culture of the late twentieth century. Orthodontists were not merely engaged in a cynical marketing ploy; they sincerely believed that good teeth contributed to a healthy psyche. In 1948 one writer argued that "the consciousness of dental beauty adds to lightness of spirit, encourages the smile of inner satisfaction, and promotes that comfortable feeling that makes life pleasant."[2] The following year, some dentists contemplated having patients with severely crooked teeth declared "dental cripples" by the state of New York, so that their orthodontic treatment could be paid for by public funds. Among the reasons cited for such a move was the stymieing impact of knowledge of one's own dental imperfection on employability and marriageability. If New York children's teeth could be improved enough to make them self-confident candidates for employment or for marriage, those children might be removed from the state's welfare rolls in adulthood.[3]

Most, however, saw orthodontics as a money-making opportunity for dentists in private practice. In the 1950s, the ADA began circulating to dentists a pamphlet entitled "Orthodontics: Questions and Answers." The pamphlet was intended for distribution by dentists seeking to bring parents up to speed with the importance of orthodontic care for their children, and thereby to drum up business for the dentists who distributed it. Consistent with the pop-psychology parlance of the day, its authors argued that "the teeth may be too conspicuous. . . . Such a condition detracts from the appearance and may produce a definite feeling of inferiority in some children and also in adults. A person's mental attitude and personal appearance can be altered."[4] This line of reasoning, familiar from its popularity early in the century, was common among orthodontists; one wrote that "a deformity of this nature is frequently associated with other problems such as: psychic disturbances, introverted personality, inferiority complex, moroseness, interference with normal employment, lack of social success, and general mental anguish."[5]

Despite their professed nostalgia for an earlier, less commercial era of dentistry, American dentists seized on orthodonture as a way of selling dental services. Unlike the sale of reparative or preventative dental care intended to treat or prevent pain, however, selling orthodontics to parents was a touchy enterprise. It required that the orthodontist point out children's aesthetic flaws without alienating them and their parents: one journal advised that orthodontists try to avoid "[pointing] out any discrepancies in a way that might make the parent feel that we think Mary is a freak of any sort."[6] Perhaps for this reason, in the early years of the orthodontics boom, orthodontists tried to emphasize the non-aesthetic benefits of orthodontics, which included more comfortable chewing, easier breathing (once the nasal passages, with the upper jaw, were appropriately widened), and teeth that were easier to keep clean and less likely to decay.

What orthodontists were really selling was an improved personal appearance—and, insofar as appearance was connected to success in business and romantic life, improved chances at both these things. The achievement of an anatomically perfect bite, which often required surgery and a lengthy period in appliances, proved an elusive dream in most cases. But increasingly, orthodontists noted that patients and families were seeking improvements that fell far short of technical correctness. They observed that "lessening of the aesthetic deficiency without a long-time effort applied to seeking perfection might suffice, or at least give satisfaction to the parents of our patients."[7] Orthodontists, patients, and their parents began to overtly declaim the benefits of aesthetic improvement with or without the technical perfection of a patient's bite. "I consider optimum facial esthetics a primary treatment goal," one dentist wrote in 1968.[8] Dentists continued to promote the health benefits of orthodontics to parents who seemed likely to pay for it on those grounds, but the major pitch more commonly had to do with appearance.

"Optimum facial esthetics" differed dramatically depending on one's personal characteristics—gender, for instance, was widely understood to be a particularly salient clinical category. Orthodontists believed that there were typically "masculine" and "feminine" tooth shapes and arrangements, which ought to be the goal of their treatment programs for young men and women, respectively. A "masculine" tooth was squarer, a "feminine" one more rounded. Some studies implicitly acknowledged the subjectivity of aesthetic appeal: for example, in one study that tried to determine the ideal relationship between teeth and the soft tissues of the face, researchers obtained their "ideal" samples by having a panel of judges "at different social status levels" choose the one hundred most attractive people (fifty men and fifty women) from a group of one thousand subjects. They then analyzed the facial angles of these "most attractive" subjects to determine what the "norms" should be.[9]

The study design seemed to concede that gender and social class could play powerful roles in shaping one's sense of what facial characteristics were beautiful. In fact, some orthodontists, by describing their work in patients' mouths as "art," implicitly admitted that there was little but the vagaries of personal taste guiding the aesthetic decisions they made.[10] However, many practitioners believed that the norms they promoted reflected a scientific basis for reaching an aesthetic judgment. Journals for orthodontists were filled with photographs and line drawings illustrating the proper angles to be formed between patients' noses, upper lips, chins, cheekbones, and teeth. Though the input of Americans from a broad range of white ethnic and socioeconomic backgrounds might be considered in determining norms, no one believed that the norms applied to individual patients ought to differ according to those patients' socioeconomic standings. While the range of possible outcomes might be limited by the patient's anatomy, or by her or his parents' willingness to pay, it was understood that orthodonture was aspirational. There was a narrow range of desirable looks, and orthodontists would choose from among them for each patient.

White orthodontists typically omitted mention of the role that race or ethnicity might play in making particular aesthetic standards desirable or achievable. Almost none frankly discussed the perceptions of race that influenced their perceptions of what was "attractive," and worth working to achieve in patients' mouths. They frequently promoted to middle-class black patients and their parents the achievement of a "more European" profile, which featured a more vertical profile line between the bottom of the nose and the edge of the chin than typically occurred naturally in black patients. One black professional from Ann Arbor, Michigan, drove his daughter into Detroit to see a black orthodontist after the white practitioners with whom he discussed his daughter's care all outlined treatment plans including the explicitly stated goal that his daughter would look "less black," which they imagined he and his child would share.[11]

The cooperation of parents was essential to orthodontists' business. Writers who described the "case presentation" phase of the dentist-patient relationship, in which the orthodontist analyzed his patients' teeth and made recommendations for their care, emphasized that it was critically important to win the confidence of both parent and child immediately. Children had to be made to feel at ease with the orthodontist, and parents had to be convinced that orthodontic care was worth their hard-earned money. Most writers recommended greeting the parent first, then the child—both with hearty handshakes and warm use of proper names.[12] Though orthodontists recognized that their child patients were likely to fear treatment, and therefore cling to their parents, most advised their peers to get the parent (usually the mother) out of the treatment room as soon as possible.[13] On the other hand, they recognized that—as one 1976 study demonstrated—parents were the ones who made decisions about whether or not to get their children's teeth fixed, and about how much money to spend in doing it. In the 1976 survey, sixty-two of eighty-nine parent-child pairs agreed that orthodontic care had been primarily the parent's idea. "This emphasizes," the study's authors concluded, "the fact that only rarely is the child consulted or involved in the decision about seeking treatment."[14] Therefore, parents had to be assiduously courted. Slowly, American parents came to accept orthodontics, and to pursue it for their children. Parents' readiness to believe that orthodontic treatment would pay off, perhaps even in dollars, was reflected in the advice that one practitioner gave to his fellows about how to discuss payment with patients' parents; he suggested that they speak of the parent's "investment" rather than of the treatment's "cost."[15]

One means of courtship was an appeal to parents' status-consciousness. Increasingly, orthodontics provided physical manifestation of one's possession of disposable income and aspirations to a "bright future." Orthodontists themselves were among the most highly compensated of dentists, and they were conscious of the advantages of class.[16] In their references to employability and marriageability, they consciously promoted aesthetic norms intended to gain for patients the financial and social stability that characterized life in the middle or upper-middle classes. In the competitive world of the postwar economic boom, aspirations of advancement were themselves an important part of class identity. In fact, some dentists commented that while they rarely belabored with patients or their parents "the social and economic values of good dental health," they did "[attempt] to subtly point out that the good results of professional care as seen by friends, coworkers and employers are as much a status symbol as the big car in the driveway."[17] Others pointed to the "desire of the American parent to do well for his children" as an important predictor of heightened demand for orthodontic services.[18] A few orthodontics researchers considered "motives involving a conspicuous achievement orientation on the part of the parents" to be a minor factor in causing a family to seek orthodontic care for one of its younger members, but others thought that such motives were so deeply rooted that they existed on an almost subconscious level. "It is very doubtful," one wrote, "that many parents are sufficiently aware of and sufficiently comfortable about their narcissistic needs and tendencies, and enough at ease about revealing their status insecurities to others, to be open about motives for orthodontic treatment that involve status and achievement issues. Conspicuous consumption is, after all, something more engaged in than readily admitted to."[19]

Aesthetic Concerns among Black Dentists and Patients

In the 1960s and 1970s, "conspicuous consumption" was not only a class but a race prerogative. Black dentists and their patients, like whites, did manifest individualist aesthetic concerns. However, the aesthetic preoccupations of black patients were much more tightly circumscribed by the underlying racial inequities in Americans' access to health care.

Black patients suffered significantly worse dental health than did whites. By 1967, the ratio of black dentists to patients had worsened: there was reportedly one dentist per 1,750 patients in the US population as a whole, but only one black dentist per 10,000 black patients.[20] The chronic shortage of black practitioners meant that black dentists filled their patient rosters without much need to promote additional services. Many of their patients would have had difficulty paying for them: though the federal government mandated certain basic services or "core components" as part of state Medicaid dental plans, the chronic underfunding of Medicaid meant that many states chose to omit these required elements, and they typically suffered no penalty for doing so.[21] Because of inadequate insurance coverage of dental care and a longstanding shortage of dentists in urban and rural areas, black patients typically waited longer than did whites to seek restorative care when it was needed. As a result, black schoolchildren suffered more untreated dental decay and more missing teeth because of decay than white children of the same ages.[22] Black dentists also had markedly less affection than did whites for the ideology of independence from government intervention that kept white dentists on the lookout for ways to promote private payment. For all these reasons, black dentists were relatively unconcerned with convincing patients to "invest" in the correction of malocclusion early in life.

Because black patients were so much more likely than whites to lose teeth, the aesthetic concern most commonly mentioned by black dentists at the end of the twentieth century was ensuring that dentures constructed to replace lost natural teeth featured gingival bases that were pigmented to match black patients' gums. In 1968, Clifton Dummett wrote that "The ever-increasing demand for a pleasing personality and good looks in every walk of life, has made people conscious of the broad black zone of pigmentation on the facial aspects of the gingivae."[23] Dummett reported that black Americans' estimation of the beauty of their mouths had increased in the wake of the "black is beautiful" movement. He argued that more work needed to be done by dentists to encourage African Americans to appreciate the natural state of their gingival tissue and to make possible the replication of racially typical gingival pigmentation in dentures. "There has been a need, from an esthetic viewpoint," he asserted, "for the development of artificial dentures which more nearly simulated the colors of the underlying tissues in instances where these tissues possessed pigmentations initially. This need for a pigmented resin for dentures in non-Caucasians cannot be underestimated."[24] Dummett commented especially on the importance of developing a pigmented resin that could be mass-produced less expensively than the hand-pigmented plastics then in use. Conscious of the growing racial disparity in wealth and in access to health care in the United States, he wrote that "economics would be a most important factor among the special people who would be using these resins."[25]

Within a decade, Dummett would have his wish: by 1971, Coe Laboratories was citing Dummett's development of a "scientific method for assessing intraoral pigmentation" as the research backing its introduction of "Natural Coe-lor" denture resin.[26] A 1972 advertisement for the product specifically mentioned the interest of "Africans, East and West Indians, Chinese, and other people of color" in replicating a "life-like" and "natural" look in their mouths.[27] In 1974, a lovely young black woman, her image captioned, "Beautiful!" gazed out from an advertisement for Hy-Pro Lucitone Fibered Dark dental resin. "True, you'll occasionally find a laboratory wizard who can take a pink denture base material and stain it to match pigmented oral tissue," the ad observed, "But it's a custom job. At a custom price. And time-consuming. Caulk's new resin shade, Hy-Pro Lucitone Fibered Dark, solves this problem for you."[28]

A series of advertisements for Bioblend porcelain teeth in the *Quarterly of the National Dental Association* struck similar notes, placing their emphasis on the importance of appearance to personal and career success, with an eye toward the cost sensitivity of older denture patients. These advertisements often appeared simultaneously in white dental journals, and usually used stock photographs of white subjects, but they demonstrated awareness of Clifton Dummett's observation that cost would be an important factor for audiences made up of people of color. A 1967 ad featured a white woman in a fur coat trying on a bracelet in a department store: "Are Bioblend Teeth just for patients who wear mink?" it asked. "No. Bioblend Teeth are for any patient who uses lipstick, goes to the hairdresser and tried her hardest to look her best. . . . In her mind the success of the denture will depend on how it looks."[29]

The ad gestured toward both the received standards of femininity that continued to be popular among black dentists with middle-class aspirations (presumably the Bioblend Teeth were not appropriate for women who did not wear lipstick) and the price sensitivity of women's interest in maintaining that standard. "The small difference in cost," the ad concluded, "is more than offset by the great difference in patient appreciation."

Advertisers in black dental journals clearly believed that a general concern for aesthetics was shared by both white and black Americans. They repeatedly chose white models for products promising aesthetically positive effects, demonstrating that they expected black dentists to adopt and promote at least some aesthetic standards in a "color-blind" fashion. Personal-care product manufacturers also perceived that black consumers, like white ones, could be sold on products using aesthetic appeals. Though the rising tide of the postwar economy lifted white Americans' boats farther and faster than it did blacks', the economic boom did leave black Americans with more disposable income than they had previously enjoyed. Racial integration and the advent of affirmative action also helped to create a class of black consumers who sought to use their purchasing power to demonstrate their class

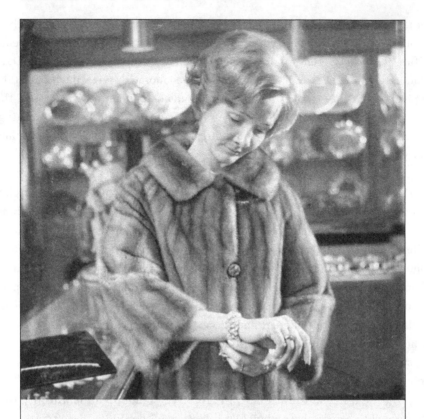

Figure 9 Advertisement for Bioblend dentures, 1967. *Quarterly of the National Dental Association* 26 (December 1967): back cover.

affiliations. Advertisements drawing on consumers' shared understanding of the importance of dental care and dental attractiveness thus appeared in black periodicals much as they did in white ones. In a 1960 *Ebony* Listerine ad titled "Protection-In-Depth," for example, a black man and woman smiled broadly as they examined fabric samples, ostensibly planning the decoration of their shared home—the ad suggested the domestic bliss that could be had by users of the product.[30] Advertisers wielded the stick as well as the carrot: in a Colgate advertisement titled "No One Wants to Go Round with Me," a young woman's brother informed her that she was unpopular because of her bad breath.[31] A series of Gleem toothpaste ads featuring prominent black Americans like jazz musician Lionel Hampton and journalist Carl Rowan appealed to the bourgeois strivings of *Ebony* readers.[32]

Advertisers clearly believed that they could assume a shared body of knowledge about bourgeois dental norms among black readers: even advertisements for products that had nothing to do with teeth reflected this conviction. A New York Life ad in 1972 pictured a cartoon black dentist and patient (the latter with a big smile) in an office setting with the caption "Your dentist can help you most if you see him regularly. The same goes for your New York Life Agent."[33] Cartoons in the magazine's long-running "Strictly for Laughs" section, too, drew upon a presumed shared experience of dentistry and its costs, and shared values about dental appearance, for their humor. In one 1975 cartoon, a black couple sat at the desk of a home improvement loan officer. The husband addressed the banker, saying "It's for my wife. I want to send her to a plastic surgeon." The cartoon signs of his wife's ostensible ugliness were her two bucked front teeth.[34] In a 1976 image, a youngster with a similar dental malady stood in front of his father (who was reading a newspaper) and mother, who had just delivered the news that the child needed to see an orthodontist. "Why does he need to have his teeth straightened?" the father asked. "According to our grocery bill, they seem to be working pretty good."[35] Both cartoons gestured not only at the currency of ideas about dentistry in the black community, but at the tension between the maintenance of a high standard of aesthetic appearance and the financial strain that black Americans frequently experienced.

The marketing of aesthetic dental interventions to black patients demonstrated dentists' and consumer-products manufacturers' understanding that race and class influenced Americans' ability to participate in the evolving norms of good looks. However, such campaigns also demonstrated that dentists and advertisers expected these new norms to be adopted as touchstones by all patients, whatever their cultural or financial circumstances. Discussion of new and higher standards of personal appearance only suggested how pervasive their influence was: even those who couldn't really afford to participate in the new norms would have to contend with them. Black dental patients experienced both financial and structural limitations on their access to new dental technologies, and to the status those technologies' use carried with them. Meanwhile, the promotion of orthodontic services, mostly to whites, worked to construct in the minds of American dentists and patients a world view in which individual markers of aspiration were also important markers of willingness to participate in the competitive world of late-twentieth-century American capitalism. Orthodontic patients, in paying for the services they received out of their pockets, visibly expressed their commitment to a politics of personal advancement by choosing to perfect their bodies. They thus also expressed some level of fealty to the entrepreneurial-capitalist vision of "Americanism" to which late-twentieth-century dentists hoped Americans would hew.

For most black dental patients, however, these visual markers of Americanness were out of financial reach. Dentists and advertisers encouraged them to pursue aesthetically pleasing mouths insofar as finances allowed, but both professionals and arbiters of popular culture sensed tension within the community of black consumers about whether, and to what extent, the new standard of personal appearance would hold sway. As they had contended with the relative scarcity of health and dental care throughout the century, black Americans coped with these aesthetic norms in varied and creative ways. Members of—and aspirants to—the black middle class clearly adopted some of the aesthetic norms being promoted most vigorously by white dentists. Working-class and rural poor blacks made use of the limited dental services offered by a disproportionately small number of black dentists. And a small but increasingly visible subset of hip-hop artists and aficionados adorned their teeth, temporarily or permanently, with precious metals and gemstones. The practice of tooth decoration was an old one: the cohort of black jazz and blues musicians who had worn gold or diamonds in their teeth in the early twentieth century understood it as a way to engage with the values of the white culture they chronicled, mourned, laughed at, and criticized in song. At the end of the century, hip-hop artists and their acolytes renewed the use of tooth decoration as a critique of whiteness, wealth, and power, and of the aesthetic norms being propagated to and by those who aspired to them.

Rob the Jewelry Store and Tell 'em "Make Me a Grill"

Early- and mid-twentieth-century traveling dentists believed that tooth decoration was a particularly fascinating vestigial element of the tribal cultures
they visited in connection with military and missionary work.[36] Most mentions of tooth decoration in the dental and popular-culture literature of the
late twentieth century also linked it—implicitly or explicitly—with the tooth-
decoration practices of some tribal peoples in Asia and Africa. Though it is not
entirely clear how tooth-decoration practices survived the journey to North
America, many early-twentieth-century black jazz and blues performers made
flamboyance, including the use of gold and diamond tooth inlays, an important part of their stage personas. Classic blues singer Ma Rainey, for example,
was renowned for her lyrical descriptions of black women's lives, particularly
their conflicted intimate relationships with men and with other women. Born
in 1886, she was described by one contemporary, pianist Mary Lou Williams,
as "loaded with real diamonds . . . her hair was wild and she had gold teeth.
What a sight! To me, as a kid, the whole thing looked and sounded weird."[37]
Ma Rainey's style of personal dress and decoration, and the attention it drew to
her lyrical message, contributed to her success as an early-twentieth-century
black feminist, highlighting—and sometimes excoriating—the racial and gender dynamics of black life in twentieth-century America.[38]

Jazz great Jelly Roll Morton likewise was renowned for his flamboyant
dress and self-decoration, including numerous pieces of diamond jewelry and
a gold-and-diamond inlay on one of his front teeth. The presence or absence
of diamonds among Morton's personal belongings served, in his own mind
and in others', as an index of his professional success. "I had plenty clothes,
plenty diamonds," he reported about one flush period.[39] Or, conversely, after
a bad run at gambling: "I had lost $20,000 and all my diamonds."[40] Though
Morton adopted his diamond tooth decoration to signal his wealth, in later
years it worked at least partly to emphasize the vanishingly small distance
between the depredations of black working-class life and his own rather tenuous financial success. At the end of his career, fortunetellers and unscrupulous music executives bilked him repeatedly, and when he died, his
diamond tooth decoration was stolen by the mortician who prepared his
body for burial.

Both Jelly Roll Morton and Ma Rainey used tooth decoration for artistic
effect, gesturing at what William Eric Perkins, describing rap, and later hip-
hop, has referred to as black popular music's "ongoing and bewildering love/

hate relationship with American society."[41] For both Rainey and Morton, gold and diamonds cemented links to the mainstream society (with its fetishism of wealth and the conspicuous display thereof) while opening opportunities for the musical critique of it. Late-twentieth-century hip-hop fashion, including rappers' penchant for quantities of gold and diamond jewelry (often fake), was similarly an attempt to "appropriate and critique through style" the wealth fetishism of white America—particularly the white America of the Reagan years. Rappers' appropriation of these fashions mocked the Western gold fetish (the source of much suffering in Africa) while affirming it.[42]

At the end of the twentieth century, black sellers and wearers of tooth jewelry explicitly emphasized its usefulness as a signifier of wealth: "People do it because they're trying to bling," reported Scott Kublin, the owner of a website that sold gold dental caps, in 2002. In an interview in the same year, rapper Darryl McDaniels of Run-DMC elaborated on what it meant to "bling" when he described why he and his fellow artists had chosen to wear such prodigious amounts of jewelry and brand-name fashion in the 1980s and 1990s. McDaniels told National Public Radio host Terry Gross: "What it actually did, [it] showed that we had money, showed that we had the big gold chain and the fancy car, and we were truly the superstars of the neighborhood. You know, if you got a big chain and the other guy don't, you *must* be doing something."[43] By the turn of the twenty-first century, hip-hop artists used gold teeth, and commentary on them, to create narrative voices that simultaneously reified wealth and status and parodied white critics' prim objections to hip-hop culture. Rapper Nelly's 2005 song "Grillz," for instance, featured the song's narrator explaining the social functions of his highly decorated teeth. "I put my money where my mouth is and bought a grill/ 20 karats 30 stacks let 'em know I'm so fo' real/ My motivation is the 30 pointers VVS/ the furniture in my mouthpiece simply symbolize success. . . . Rob the jewelry store and tell 'em 'Make me a grill.'"[44]

Dentists and pop-culture commentators grasped that hip-hop artists intended to offer comment on the tight connection between dental appearance and social and economic success. But white media coverage of tooth decoration at the end of the twentieth century erred in taking hip-hop's fetishization of wealth too seriously. It responded to the literal claims of hip-hop, and not to the broader critiques of white culture often being levied. Such coverage prudishly argued that the appearance of wealth associated with tooth decoration was misleading, and disparaged the practice on the grounds that it made people with gold teeth look scary and unemployable. Tooth decoration was linked to blackness, poverty, and bad judgment in a number of high-profile, and widely reprinted, articles in the late 1990s and beyond. One item, originally published in the *Houston Chronicle* and reprinted in the *Raleigh News and Observer*, featured a full-color photo of a black man with gold dental work: the headline on the piece read "Gold in the Mouth, but None in the Pocket: Employers Turned Off by Youth Fad."[45] A career counselor advised one Houston woman to have the gold decorations in her teeth removed, and a local dentist recruited a sponsor to pay the costs of replacing the gold tooth with a "normal-looking cap."[46] The director of the Texas School of Business told the reporter who interviewed her about the case that "gold is a barrier. People make instant judgments when they meet someone."[47]

The safety of tooth decoration was mentioned in only four paragraphs at the end of a forty-one-paragraph article. Other white media coverage emphasized the danger of dental decay and erosion caused by tooth decoration, implicitly or explicitly accusing those with gold teeth of bad judgment or inadequate concern for long-term dental health. One item in New York's *Newsday* characterized gold caps as "a dentist's nightmare. They are placed directly over the tooth by a jeweler and lack the careful fitting of crowns prepared by licensed dentists."[48] The article mentioned Brooklyn dentist Ann Linton, a black woman, for her campaign to stamp out the practice of tooth decoration among the city's youth. "She has handed out fliers at health fairs and at events that draw large black youth populations," the article concluded.[49] Other observers of the practice went farther: in Louisiana, State Representative Ed Murray, a Democrat, proposed a bill that "would make it a crime for a dentist to put gold teeth, fillings or crowns in the mouths of persons under 18 without the consent of their parents." To the *New Orleans Times-Picayune*, Murray described the bill as "an effort to keep dentists from exploiting young people trying to follow a fad."[50] Such coverage capitalized on the popular understanding of African American youth as status-seeking, uneducated, perhaps even anti-intellectual—in short, as uncritical thinkers, and as slow responders to scientific logic about the wisdom of altering one's teeth.

Though white people wore gold tooth decorations, most journalistic coverage of the trend cast it as exclusively black. White dentists who confronted gold dental work in the mouths of black patients struggled to contend with the conflicting demands of cultural sensitivity and professional orthodoxy about aesthetics. An article in the *Atlanta Journal and Constitution* concluded with Dr. Richard Smith, of the Georgia Dental Association, making a weak gesture in the direction of cultural relativism. "Any of the reputable dentists I know wouldn't do it," he said. "Cosmetically, I don't see where it has a place. But in a certain culture, if people want to do it, I can't say it's not valid."[51] An editorial in the *Baltimore Sun* commented more directly on the racialized perception of gold teeth in black mouths by a white audience. Its author observed the irony of a recent item on gold caps having appeared next to an article on the "preponderance of black students who get suspended from public school."[52] "We're not inferring that white teachers see a black student with a gold tooth and haul him to the principal's office," the article cautioned, "but you can't deny cultural differences based on race. You see someone wearing an adornment that seems peculiar, affecting a machismo that's intimidating, and the relationship descends from there."[53] The editorial argued that the "cultural difference" of black students' preference for gold dental adornment, and white teachers' aversion to that aesthetic, was "based on race." Gold teeth, its author felt, had become so strongly associated with blackness—and therefore, in the minds of white teachers, with criminality and the need for discipline—that dental "adornments" served primarily to alienate black students from the white mainstream. The idea that news items like the one titled "Gold in the Mouth, but None in the Pocket" might have helped to create or reinforce the association of gold teeth with blackness, poverty, and shiftlessness in the minds of newspaper readers apparently did not occur to him.

The argument that children, in particular, needed to be protected from bad decision-making about dental health and personal appearance recapitulated one of the central themes of twentieth-century American thinking about community responsibility for individuals' dental health. Free enterprise, most agreed, had to be allowed to flourish—but the young, who could not be expected to make good decisions for themselves (or to be able to access dental care or services consistent with the good decisions they might happen to make) usually deserved government protection from the hazards of the marketplace. Most tooth decoration at the end of the twentieth century was done by jewelers who were not trained in dentistry. The rare coverage of dentists who did install tooth decorations—thereby, presumably, decreasing the risk that they would damage the natural teeth—treated the practitioners as delusional: the *Wall Street Journal*, profiling the career of white "Rapper Dentist Daddy" Ronald Cunning, quoted rapper C-Murder ("a 26-year-old New Orleans rap artist [also known as Corey Miller, 'but you can call me Murder']") commenting that Cunning was "the real."[54] The article initially conceded that there might be some broader cultural point being made by tooth decoration, describing gold and diamond tooth implants as "long a fashion accessory in certain African-American circles of the Deep South."[55] But the narrator made both C-Murder and his dentist Cunning into figures of comic attention rather than studied respect. Cunning lacked even the cultural knowledge necessary to identify the format of his patients' products (he called CDs "little records"), naively came to the conclusion that his replacement of C-Murder's healthy natural teeth with gold and diamond crowns looked "just beautiful," and said that notorious rap artist Eminem (at the time, much discussed in the news for his lyrical threats to kill his mother and his ex-wife, Kim Mathers) "seem[ed] like a real nice guy." C-Murder, on the other hand, planned to memorialize Dr. Cunning in an upcoming album: "It'll be real clean, of course," the article concluded.[56]

The article's author clearly conceived of C-Murder's choice to decorate his teeth as a sign of his individual aspirations and commitments, which the piece sought to portray as antithetical to the values of *Wall Street Journal* readers. The disparaging tone the writer adopted in this effort contrasted dramatically with the two-line ad for a Lexus automobile published in the *Wall Street Journal* not long before. Like the article, the Lexus ad, pairing the sentence "Naturally, all our kids wear braces," with a smaller-font rendering of the Lexus motto ("The Relentless Pursuit of Perfection"),[57] drew on values that Lexus marketers assumed were shared by *Wall Street Journal* readers. Straight teeth—teeth, in fact, that were visibly in the process of being straightened—were understood to be an important (even "natural") marker of high social and economic status. Children and automobiles, as appropriate sites for the affectionate display of conspicuous consumption, were also both recognized as sites for the demonstration of one's consumer capacity—and, thereby, one's standing in American society. "The Relentless Pursuit of Perfection" was understood to be an aspiration properly shared not only by Japanese automobile manufacturers, but by upper- and upper-middle-class American parents—and by orthodontists.

Like the profile of Dr. Cunning and C-Murder, the ad implicitly assumed that its readers shared, and regarded as important, values about the appearance of one's teeth. The editors of, and advertisers in, the *Wall Street Journal* clearly believed that readers would understand orthodontics and tooth decoration to be completely unrelated—that, in fact, readers would regard the values they represented as being in opposition to one another. The Lexus ad argued for a class consciousness of one's children's teeth as a marker of social standing. C-Murder's gold grill, by contrast, was portrayed as demonstrating his bizarre lack of awareness that such consciousness was desirable.

The belief that C-Murder's and Lexus's target audiences were living in different cultural, esthetic, and moral worlds was certainly widespread, but it was, in important ways, inaccurate. Late-twentieth-century Americans' renowned obsession with the straightness and whiteness of their teeth was—as is true of almost any expensive hobby—a product of ideas about race and class, and the way those ideas influenced aesthetic values. For the white dentists who promoted orthodontics, the specialty represented an opportunity to emphasize the American values of ambition and individual responsibility. For white commentators on tooth decoration, the racialized attribution of poverty, sloth, and bad taste to those who decorated their teeth with gold and diamonds helped to reinforce the idea that a mouth full of clean, healthy, straight teeth was an appropriate aspiration for Americans at the turn of the twenty-first century. But black Americans who decorated their teeth weren't ignorant of these norms: rather, they sought to challenge them. Tooth decoration critiqued the prevailing construction of the mouth as a place where an American might—and ought to—demonstrate high social standing, good judgment, and easy access to high-quality dental care.

Epilogue

"Brits resort to pulling own teeth," trumpeted CNN.com in October 2007. The article went on to explain that a shortage of dentists in the National Health Service was driving patients to take treatment into their own hands. "I took most of my teeth out in the shed with pliers," one unhappy interviewee said. "I have one to go."[1] In June 2008, the television channel BBC America began running a documentary called *Britain's Worst Teeth*, which emphasized the two-year wait for some kinds of dental procedures in the United Kingdom. Scary reports from locales in which dental care was inaccessible—particularly because of the widely scorned insufficiencies of programs of social insurance—reinforced the consensus among American dentists and patients that bad dental care, and the poor personal appearance that could result from it, were horrors to be avoided at all costs. The belief that dentistry was important, and that it ought to be delivered more or less in the way that dentists said it should, represented a signal success for organized American dentistry in the twentieth century.

Consumer-products advertising certainly helped to promote the new aesthetic norms to which patients and prospective patients were increasingly expected to adhere. Likewise, the surging popularity of "reality" television programs encouraged Americans to think of themselves as persons constantly on the verge of great notoriety, who needed to maintain Hollywood standards of personal beauty at all times. *American Idol* winner Carrie Underwood, an exemplar of this imminent visibility, told *Us Weekly* in 2008: "I like my teeth. Sometimes I wonder if my orthodontist realizes how important he was."[2]

Patients' increasing demand for aesthetic services reflected their rising disposable incomes, their freedom from the dental decay and pain that had been partially alleviated by fluoride, and an escalating tendency to regard personal style as a statement of one's political, economic, and social affiliations and aspirations. But the most powerful and intentional force militating in the direction of the new norms of dental appearance was the activism of American dentists themselves. In the late twentieth and early twenty-first centuries, dentists fearing real and imagined threats to their incomes and professional autonomy sought to inculcate Americans with an aspirational vision of dental health and appearance that depended on extensive individual investment of time and money into dental treatment, and they were largely successful in doing so.

As a result, the market for aesthetic dental services like orthodonture and tooth whitening ballooned. "A trip to the dentist used to mean standard cleaning, drilling and filling," explained one *Newsweek* writer in 1998, "But thanks to fluoridated water and better dental hygiene, Americans' oral health has vastly improved. Now dentists—drilling for new revenue sources—are mingling words like 'self-esteem' with 'gingivitis.' Like surgery, dentistry is going cosmetic."[3] In 2005, the "consumer advisor" for the American Dental Association estimated that dentists were performing "twice as many cosmetic procedures as they were just three years ago . . . and companies have sprung up to offer special financing for those who'd like to remodel their mouths."[4] Popular news sources reporting on the trend identified it as a new and uniquely American one: "With the vast majority of celebrities sporting blinding-white smiles, and shows like 'Extreme Makeover' bringing da Vinci veneers to Everyman, Americans have grown tooth-obsessed," *Newsweek* proclaimed in 2005.

Americans' worldwide reputation as a people possessed of unique fastidiousness about the appearance of their teeth was not as new as media coverage made it seem. In the late 1960s, for instance, renowned British cellist Jacqueline DuPre ranted to her sister Hilary about a characteristic she had noted in her American audiences: "I'm fascinated by American mouths. . . . Rows of perfect teeth, set in a hideous grin, and a gushing 'aren't we pals' expression."[5] DuPre's comments would be echoed three decades later by the London-dwelling musician who said he could tell when he was performing in the United States by the "piano teeth" in the audience.[6] The tone of comment on Americans' uniquely perfect teeth reflected political and cultural conditions that changed over time. In the terror-war climate of the post-9/11 era, for instance, one urban legend suggested that having distinctively American teeth might pose a risk to either personal safety or national security. "A few months ago I was reading an article about the structuring of overseas US intelligence," one blogger wrote. "There was a piece about a new recruit who showed up, accompanied by his blinding white smile. A seasoned veteran took a look at his pearly whites and told him he'd have to put a hammer to his dental work before he could accompany him on his missions . . . his brilliant, perfect dental work would have them identified and killed immediately."[7]

In general, however, popular commentators on Americans' internationally renowned dental obsession at the turn of the twenty-first century figured it as a combined product of historically unequalled national prosperity and the perennial American propensity to pursue all opportunities to their farthest extremes of fruition. Comedy, in particular, depended on these associations for its currency. In April 2003, for instance, the satirical newspaper *The Onion* reported that "US Dentists Can't Make Nation's Teeth Any Damn Whiter." "The typical ADA dentist," the health-column send-up informed readers, "is irked by customers who come in for routine bleaching and leave disappointed because 'their teeth don't inflict retinal damage when you look directly into them. . . . When someone creates a better tooth-whitening procedure, we'll slap an 'ultra' on it and get it out on the market as fast as the FDA allows. Until then, be happy with what you have. Americans really need to learn to live with almost-total perfection."[8] In 2007, the comic strip "Bizarro" featured a woman whose teeth were emitting a blinding glare telling a man that "Whitening strips are SO last year. Now it's all about halogen implants."[9]

The comic trope of the tooth-obsessed American—and her perennial antagonist, the Briton heedless of the importance of good dentistry—extended far beyond the funny pages. In a 1993 episode of *The Simpsons*, for instance, Springfield dentist Dr. Wolf intimidated young patient Ralph Wiggum into committing to brush his teeth more often by showing him the *Big Book of British Smiles*.[10] Comedian Mike Myers's series of *Austin Powers* films repeatedly used the eponymous hero's teeth as indicators of both historical time and Powers's nationality. When British hipster/ international spy Austin Powers first burst into theaters in 1997, he had just been reanimated after a thirty-year stay in cryogenic storage. His love interest, played by the famously gorgeous Elizabeth Hurley, complained to her mother about Powers's crooked, cruddy teeth, only to be told that "in Britain, in the sixties, you could be a sex symbol and still have bad teeth!" Powers subsequently saved humanity from the machinations of his aptly named nemesis, Dr. Evil, by swinging over a moat on a rope of dental floss conveniently produced by the hygiene-conscious Hurley at the pivotal moment. In the second film in the trilogy, in which the action shifted back and forth between the UK in 1969 and the US in 1999, Powers's teeth—crooked and stained in the former, and straight and shiny in the latter—were even more important markers of both modernity and nation, letting viewers know *when*, as well as *where*, Powers was. After preventing Dr. Evil from annihilating Washington, DC, with a blast from a giant laser, Powers was rewarded with the affection of another love interest—a blonde, blue-eyed American CIA agent played by Heather Graham. Her romantic capitulation to Powers as the film closed and Lenny Kravitz's funk-infused version of the Guess Who classic "American Woman" played communicated that Powers's straight, shining teeth were part of a uniquely American package of social and sexual success. Bad teeth, the films indicated, were an outdated British phenomenon; good teeth were modern, American, and heroic.

In real life, political gadfly Christopher Hitchens, a Briton who was naturalized in the United States in April 2007, described his acquisition of new dental veneers that fall as "part of my new passport to Americanization." His dentist's colleague, he reported, came by to see Hitchens's teeth before the procedure began, because he "wanted to see with his own eyes that my teeth were really as 'British' as they looked in the 'before' photograph." Hitchens's six hours in the dental chair not only took away the "stains and the shame" of his native dentition; they also provided him with an opportunity to appreciate the tightening link between personal aesthetic aspiration and access to the luxury and the pampering afforded to the very rich. During his treatment, Hitchens listened to music from the dentist's "massively accoutred Sonos sound system . . . [and] a foot masseur was thoughtfully provided to alleviate the tedium."[11]

The widespread adoption of the aesthetic norms promoted by dentists reflected patients' genuine interests in personal appearance. As Hitchens's reference to "stains and shame" suggested, though, it also helped to create a climate of aesthetic expectation that was stifling for the many who did not, or could not, conform. Reflecting on the chronic undersupply of basic dental care in rural Kentucky, *New York Times* writer Ian Urbina reported that Barbourville dentist Edwin E. Smith "has seen the shame of a 14-year-old girl who would not lift her head because she had lost most of her teeth from malnutrition." The director of an employment placement program in Appalachia similarly challenged Urbina: "Try finding work when you're in your 30s or 40s and you're missing front teeth."[12]

Heightened aesthetic expectations themselves combined with the popular association of bad dental health with tobacco and methamphetamine use, malnutrition, and poverty made unattractive teeth a source of humiliation. The final link in the chain of association was the shared belief that all of these characteristics—ugliness, bad health choices, and personal impoverishment—could be correctly attributed to a failure of personal ambition. The social prohibition on openly admitting that one judged acquaintances by their appearance—always more honored in the breach than in the observance—was quickly being erased, and in ways that made refusal to engage with the new dental aesthetic norms increasingly untenable. In 2003, *New York Times* writer Natalie Angier conducted an "informal e-mail tooth survey of twenty-seven colleagues and friends [asking] . . . whether they noticed other people's teeth." Two-thirds told Angier that they did. One historian reported to Angier: "I'm put off by bad teeth. They give a low-life impression. Dental elitism, that's me."[13] Individuals' failures to maintain good dental health and appearance were commonly understood to represent lack of personal drive or efficacy, normalizing the pursuit of good looks. In 2008, 60 percent of respondents to a survey on the website of the upscale men's magazine *Best Life* said that they considered tooth whitening "normal"; only 6 percent called it "excessively vain."[14] People with bad teeth could be safely judged—or, as in the Myers films, mocked.

Dentists' moves to promote patient aspiration to high aesthetic standards had an impact not only on the patients who adopted or contended with those norms, but on the larger cultural, professional, and political worlds of which dentists were a part. As they abandoned their previous commitment to public-health strategies to lift health standards on a community basis, dentists also jettisoned the notion that Americans—and particularly wealthy, well-educated Americans—had any obligation to work for social change. Dentists' resistance to a national program of dental insurance meant that federal funding for dental care ultimately occurred through the chronically underfunded Medicaid system administered by individual states. Though the federal government set minimum standards for state dental plans, many states failed to meet the required thresholds, and many dentists chose not to accept Medicaid recipients as patients at all, leaving poor adults and children without access to needed services.[15] In Maryland, for example, only 900 of the 5,500 dentists in the state accepted Medicaid in 2007.[16]

Early in the twenty-first century, the results of these inequities in access began to show in Americans' mouths and bodies. For the first time in fifty years, the CDC announced in 2007, the percentage of Americans with untreated cavities was rising.[17] That year in Maryland, twelve-year-old Deamonte Driver died of meningitis after a tooth abscess spread to his brain. The *Washington Post* reported that Driver's mother, Alyce, had experienced extreme difficulty keeping her children enrolled in Medicaid and finding a dentist who would provide services under the plan. Because of the resultant delays in his care, her son was hospitalized for two weeks and underwent brain surgery costing approximately $250,000 before he died.[18]

The *New York Times* reported that despite the large unmet need for basic dental services, and the excessive health care spending that could result after lapses in essential care, the ADA continued to oppose increasing the size of the pool of dental health care providers, agitating against the opening of new dental schools and the training of advanced-practice dental hygienists. The ADA's opposition, news coverage hypothesized, was directly linked to dentists' interest in maintaining their personal incomes. "Dental fees have risen much faster than inflation," the *Times* article concluded. "In real dollars, the cost of the average dental procedure rose 25 percent from 1996 to 2004."[19] Dentists, the *Times* said, were reaping enormous financial rewards for their diligence in protecting the elite status of the profession: "[Their] incomes have grown faster than that of the typical American and the incomes of medical doctors. Formerly poor relations to physicians, American dentists in general practice made an average salary of $185,000 in 2004. . . . Dental surgeons and orthodontists average more than $300,000 annually."[20]

Some dentists who responded to the report in the *Times'* editorial pages pointed to the need for an increase in Medicaid, State Children's Health Insurance Program, and insurance reimbursements in order to provide dentists with an incentive to provide more basic dental care. But one letter writer provided a pessimistic satire of what could be accomplished through government intervention with his proposal for a "No Dental Patient Left Behind plan." He imagined that such a program might ape the worst features of the famously imprecise testing and "accountability" measures introduced into Title I of the Elementary and Secondary Education Act (popularly known as "No Child Left Behind") when it was reauthorized in 2001. In the letter writer's dystopian vision, "All American residents will be assigned to a public dental clinic, which will be financed primarily by local property taxes. That will ensure that the quality of dental care available in every jurisdiction will be roughly proportional to real estate values. . . . Dentists' renewed commitment to eradicate tooth decay, the revealing light cast by systematic testing, and the superior management that will come with state takeovers will combine to make America decay-free by 2014, at which time we will look back on the benighted era of c. 2007 with disbelief," he concluded.[21] The contrast between his cynical skepticism of socially shared solutions and the optimism that had undergirded the Cleveland and Bridgeport dental hygiene campaigns early in the twentieth century could hardly have been starker.

The anxieties about professional status and autonomy that had animated many of dentists' behaviors throughout the 1900s drove their desires to keep the pool of dental care providers small in the twenty-first century. Complaints and concerns about insurance programs and their effects on dental practice featured prominently in dentists' responses to criticism from outside the profession. Most of all, the rightward political shift that had prompted dentists' late-century skepticism of "big government" and their turn away from public health solutions continued to shape their sense of what was possible, and desirable, for American dental patients. This rightward shift in dentists' thinking mirrored the increasingly entrenched American belief that comparatively few individual health expenses ought to be socially shared, and that individuals who failed to provide adequately for their own health expenses could be ignored or reviled with impunity. The climate produced by this confluence of forces helped to ensure the continued power and prestige of dentists, but it also guaranteed that inequity in access to dental care would continue, increasing the distance between Americans and the dream of the American mouth.

Notes

Introduction

1. Lexus advertisement, *Wall Street Journal*, Wednesday, October 27, 1999.
2. Janet Carlson Freed, "Word of Mouth: Cosmetic Treatments for Teeth," *Town & Country* 152 (August 1998): 54.
3. Elizabeth Hayt, "Blinding Them with Smiles," *New York Times*, September 18, 2000.
4. Ibid.
5. "Dental and Oral Conditions of Recruits," *Dental Cosmos* (September 1916): 1071–1075.
6. A. Lehrmann, "A Few Words about the Practice of Dentistry Here with That in Russia," *Western Dental Journal* 21 (January 1907): 10.
7. For a short description of the effects of the Harrison Act and its enforcement, see Margaret Battin et al., *Drugs and Justice: Seeking a Consistent, Coherent, Comprehensive View* (New York: Oxford University Press, 2008), 34.
8. See, for example, Kathy Peiss, *Cheap Amusements: Working Women and Leisure in Turn-of-the-Century New York* (Philadelphia: Temple University Press, 1986).
9. Elizabeth Giangrego, "The Life and Times of Painless Parker," as published by the Pierre Fauchard Academy on its website, www.fauchard.org/inquiries/museum/07/PP/index.htm (accessed May 19, 2008).
10. Malvin Ring, *Dentistry: An Illustrated History* (St. Louis: Mosby, 1985), 4.
11. James Wynbrandt, *The Excruciating History of Dentistry* (New York: St. Martin's Press, 1998), 146
12. Frank Norris, *McTeague: A Story of San Francisco* (1899; repr., New York: Penguin Books, 1982), passim.
13. The figure of McTeague played powerfully in dentists' minds as an example of inadequate ambition. One writer summoned up the character to dismiss other dentists who failed to adapt to new social and economic conditions this way: "Standards had changed. McTeague's inability to grasp the fact of change, to reconcile himself to its logical inevitability, and to adapt himself to a new order of events, far removed from the grooves in which he had spent his daily life for fifteen years, is strikingly comparable, it seems to me, to the perturbed effusions concerning social changes today. Too many of us have believed we have made vocational adjustments whereas in reality we have merely fitted ourselves into grooves . . ." "E.H.D," "Beneath It All," *Dental Digest* 40 (August 1934): 281.
14. On the process of raising educational standards within medicine, see Kenneth Ludmerer, *Learning to Heal: The Development of American Medical Education* (Baltimore: Johns Hopkins University Press, 1985). In dentistry, see Norman Gevitz, "Autonomous Profession or Medical Specialty: The Stomatological Movement and American Dentistry," *Bulletin of the History of Medicine* 62 (1988): 410.
15. In 1918, a B'nai Brith survey suggested that 23.4 percent of all dental students in the United States were Jewish (Hasia Diner, *In the Almost Promised Land: American Jews and Blacks, 1915–1935* [Westport, Conn.: Greenwood Press, 1977], 5). But,

as Edward Halperin has demonstrated elsewhere, the statistical overrepresentation of Jews in professional schools in the 1900s and 1910s upset Protestant university leaders, who responded by instituting quotas on Jewish admission in the 1920s. See Halperin, "The Jewish Problem in US Medical Education, 1920–1955," *Journal of the History of Medicine and the Allied Sciences* 56 (2001): 140–167.

16. The National Dental Association renamed itself the American Dental Association in 1921. Black dentists later adopted the name the white organization had abandoned; their organizations were affiliates of the larger entity, the National Dental Association (NDA).

17. C. N. Johnson, "Stomatology or Dentistry?" *Journal of the American Dental Association* 13 (1926): 371–372, as cited in Norman Gevitz, "Autonomous Profession or Medical Specialty: The Stomatological Movement and American Dentistry," *Bulletin of the History of Medicine* 62 (1988): 407–428.

18. Amy Green, "Tooth and Nails," *Southwest Airlines Spirit* (in-flight magazine), August 2005, 82.

19. On homes and other consumer goods, see, for example, Lizabeth Cohen, *A Consumer's Republic: The Politics of Mass Consumption in Postwar America* (New York: Knopf, 2003), and Jeffrey Hornstein, *A Nation of Realtors: A Cultural History of the Twentieth-Century American Middle Class* (Durham, N.C.: Duke University Press, 2005). On bodies, see Elizabeth Haiken, *Venus Envy: A History of Cosmetic Surgery* (Baltimore: Johns Hopkins University Press, 1997), and Kathy Peiss, *Hope in a Jar: The Making of America's Beauty Culture* (New York: Metropolitan Books, 1998).

Chapter 1 — American Dental Hygiene

1. "Oral Hygiene to Become a National Movement at Cleveland, Ohio, March 18, 1910: President Taft and the Governors of the United States to Be Invited to Attend the Opening," *The Dental Brief* 15 (March 1910): 212.

2. W. G. Ebersole, "Report of the Proposed Dental, Educational, and Hygienic Work in the Cleveland Public Schools," as published by *The Dental Brief* 15 (March 1910): 215. Ebersole, a Cleveland native, was the chairman of the National Dental Association's Committee on Oral Hygiene. I have indicated when I am citing a paper initially presented in public and later reprinted by a professional journal by describing it "as published by": comments on public presentations are listed, commenter's name first, followed by "comments on" (or "commenting on") and the rest of the citation.

3. W. H. Elson, "Address of Welcome," as published by *The Dental Brief* 15 (May 1910): 390.

4. G. C. Ashmun, "Opening of the National Campaign on Oral Hygiene," as published by *The Dental Brief* 15 (May 1910): 389.

5. Henry C. Muckley, "Our Interest in the Work," as published by *The Dental Brief* 15 (May 1910): 394.

6. "The Marion School Squad," *Oral Hygiene* 1 (July 1911): 506

7. Ibid., 506.

8. The logic behind the decision to award this financial incentive on Christmas is difficult to discern. It may have reflected the planners' own sense that special financial considerations, like employment bonuses, were most properly awarded during the Christian holiday season—or it may have represented an explicit attempt at religious and/or cultural conversion. The school dental nurse, in her

report on the hygiene activities she carried out with the students, listed the Jewish High Holy Days together with electrical service outages as causes of slowed progress on the project. "Report on the Activities of the Dental Nurse in Marion School, Cleveland, Ohio," *Dental Digest* 16 (February 1911): 144.

9. Ibid., 143.

10. William G. Ebersole, "The Human Mouth and Its Relation to the Health, Strength, and Beauty of the Nation," *The Dental Cosmos* 53, date unknown: 798.

11. Cordelia O'Neill, "Oral Hygiene: An Important Factor in the Conservation of the Child," *Oral Hygiene* 1 (October 1919): 736.

12. Ibid., 734.

13. "Report of Activities," *Dental Digest* 16 : 144.

14. Lillian Cohen, "What the Marion School Squad Did for Me," *Dental Digest* 17 (September 1911): 508.

15. "Incorrigible Pupils Now Well Behaved," *The Dental Brief* 16 (June 1911): 439.

16. Lillian Gottfreid, "What the Marion School Squad Did for Me," *Dental Digest* 17 (September 1911): 506.

17. On the ideology of the germ and the public health campaigns that resulted, see Nancy Tomes, *The Gospel of Germs: Men, Women, and the Microbe in American Life* (Cambridge: Harvard University Press, 1998), and Richard Meckel, *Save the Babies: American Public Health Reform and the Prevention of Infant Mortality, 1850–1929* (Baltimore: Johns Hopkins University Pres, 1990). On school medical inspection programs, see Howard Markel, "For the Welfare of Children: The Origins of the Relationship between US Public Health Workers and Pediatricians," in Howard Markel and Alexandra Minna Stern, eds., *Formative Years: Children's Health in the United States, 1880–2000* (Ann Arbor: University of Michigan Press, 2002), especially pages 57–61.

18. William Belcher, "God's Poor and a Few 'Poor Devils': An Address on Free Dispensary Service," as published by *The Dental Cosmos* 52 (April 1910): 450. A dentist from the US Indian Service Field Dental Corps made a similar point with respect to dental service the government provided for the estimated 300,000 Natives then living on reservations: "This requires the annual expenditure of a large appropriation having for its ultimate end the preparation of the remnants of this once strong and vigorous race for the privileges of citizenship," he wrote. Fdo. Rodriguez, "The United States Indian Service Field Dental Corps: A New Field of Activity in Which Physician, Dentist and Teacher Collaborate," as published by *Dental Items of Interest* 39 (May 1917): 364.

19. This logic guided the spending of wealthy philanthropists like Carnegie, who spent millions on libraries and educational institutions during the same period, but who typically refused to endow a library until its home community or institution had raised as much money as Carnegie himself was asked to donate. On the conditions for Carnegie's endowments, see Donna K. Cohen, "Andrew Carnegie and Academic Library Philanthropy: the Case of Rollins College," *Libraries and Culture* 35 (Summer 2000): 389–415. Even the physical layout of the Carnegie libraries, which innovated in making open stacks of books available to the public, was intended to promote self-sufficiency. See Abigail A. van Slyck, " 'The Utmost Amount of Effectiv [sic] Accommodation': Andrew Carnegie and the Reform of the American Library," *Journal of the Society of Architectural Historians* 50 (December 1991): 359–383.

20. Belcher, "God's Poor," *The Dental Cosmos* 52: 456.

21. George Hardisty, "Oral Hygiene in Our Public Schools," as published by *The Dental Cosmos* 43 (August 1901): 951.

22. George Edwin Hunt, "Oral Hygiene," as published by *Dental Digest* 11 (July 1905): 653. Hunt would go on to become editor of his own journal, the Indianapolis-based *Oral Hygiene*, in 1911.

23. William Trueman, commenting on Alphonso Irwin, "Oral Prophylaxis as a Municipal Problem," as published by *Dental Brief* 18 (September 1913): 633.

24. O'Neill, "Oral Hygiene: An Important Factor," *Oral Hygiene* 1: 734. George Edwin Hunt, the editor of *Oral Hygiene*, wrote: "And mind you, Cleveland has had medical inspection of its school children for the past three years, so the physician has had his 'whack' at them before the dentists came along" (George Edwin Hunt, "The Marion School Squad," *Oral Hygiene* 1 [July 1911]: 507).

25. "A 'Mischief-Breeding Neglect,'" *The Dental Cosmos* 44 (March 1902): 296.

26. "Iconoclast," "Dentistry—Duty and Opportunity," *The Dental Brief* 14 (September 1909): 642.

27. "Report of Activities," *Dental Digest* 16: 144–145.

28. Ebersole, "The Human Mouth," *The Dental Cosmos* 53, 794.

29. Ibid., 797.

30. Charlotte Fitzhugh Morris, "Oral Hygiene at Locust Point," *Dental Digest* 24 (1), January 1918, 3.

31. See, for instance, Selma Berrol, "Immigrant Children at School, 1880–1940: A Child's-Eye View," in Elliott West and Paula Petrik, eds., *Small Worlds: Children and Adolescents in America, 1850–1950* (Lawrence: University Press of Kansas, 1992), 42–60. On Italian immigrants' attitudes toward prolonged schooling, see Stephen Lassonde, "Should I Go, or Should I Stay?: Adolescence, School Attainment, and Parent-Child Relations in Italian Immigrant Families of New Haven, 1900–1940," *History of Education Quarterly* 38 (Spring 1998): 37–60. On Jewish mothers' attitudes toward American medical care, see Jacquelyn Litt, "Mothering, Medicalization, and Jewish Identity, 1928–1940," *Gender and Society* 10 (April 1996): 185–198.

32. These notices were often produced by state or local dental societies and distributed either under the byline of an individual dentist or anonymously. A local newspaper editor in Crawfordsville, Indiana, objected to both the notices themselves (which he considered unethical attempts to bilk newspaper editors out of advertising space) and to the practice of publishing them without bylines, "indicating that it is the purpose of the society to deceive the public as well as the publisher." The editor proposed that dentists advertise openly instead. (George Edwin Hunt, "The Public Be Damned," *Oral Hygiene* 1 [August 1911]: 592.)

33. Russell Cool, "Popular Dissemination of Dental Knowledge," as published by *The Pacific Stomatological Gazette* 4 (August 1896): 349.

34. J. Percell Corley, "Popular Dental Education," as published by *The Dental Cosmos* 43 (January 1901): 33.

35. C. E. Post, commenting on Frank Platt, "Dentists as Public Educators," as published by *The Pacific Stomatological Gazette* 4 (October 1896): 446.

36. E. M. Wolfe, commenting on H. H. Harrison, "Popular Dental Education," as published by *The Ohio Dental Journal* 16 (August 1896): 381.

37. On human waste and insects, see Tomes, *The Gospel of Germs*.

38. George Edwin Hunt, "The Economic Value of Clean Mouths," as published by *Oral Hygiene* 2 (November 1912): 861.

39. Richard Grady, "Cooperation of the Public Schools in Teaching 'Good Teeth, Good Health,'" as published by *The American Journal of Dental Science* 35 (August 1904): 143.

40. Mrs. Hubert W. Hart, "Working Out the Details of a Preventive Dental Clinic for School Children," as published by *The Dental Cosmos* 57 [October 1915]: 1129.

41. Hardisty, "Oral Hygiene in Our Public Schools," 951.

42. Alfred Fones, "A Plan that Solves the Fundamental Problem in School Hygiene," as published by *Oral Hygiene* 4 (January 1914): 10.

43. E. Burton Newell, "A General Appeal to Citizens For Cooperation In Restoring to Health the Diseased Mouths of Our School Children," as published by *The Dental Brief* 17 (September 1912): 704. On "schoolroom poisoning" as described by school medical inspectors, see Richard Meckel, "Going to School, Getting Sick: The Social and Medical Construction of School Diseases in the Late Nineteenth Century," in Markel and Stern, eds, *Formative Years*, especially pages 195–198.

44. Cool, *The Pacific Stomatological Gazette* 4: 346.

45. "The First 'Mouth Hygiene' Mass Meeting in History Held at Convention Hall, Rochester, NY," *The Dental Brief* 16 (January 1911): 61.

46. Cool, *Pacific Stomatological Gazette* 4: 347. For more on gold dental work and dentists' beliefs about it, see chapter 7.

47. Richard Grady, "Oral Hygiene for the School Boy and Girl," as published by *The Dental Cosmos* 46 (February 1904): 133.

48. Ibid., 134–135.

49. "National Dental Association Committee on Oral Hygiene in Public Schools: An Appeal for Co-Operation," *The Dental Cosmos* 44 (April 1902): 401.

50. See, for example, " 'Mouth Hygiene' Mass Meeting," 60–63, and Arthur H. Merritt, "The Dental Clinics of the Children's Aid Society," *Oral Hygiene* 1 (December 1911): 911–918.

51. "The Forsyth Dental Infirmary for Children," *The Dental Brief* 16 (April 1911): 266.

52. Ibid., 264

53. "Dedication of the Forsyth Dental Infirmary," *Oral Hygiene* 5 (January 1915): 15.

54. Ibid., 18.

55. Ibid., 20.

56. Ibid., 21.

57. Ibid., 21.

58. Ibid., 13.

59. Ibid., 14.

60. Ibid., 15.

61. Ibid., 17.

62. Ibid., 21.

63. George Wood Clapp, "The Rise and Fall of Oral Hygiene in Bridgeport (First Article)," *Dental Digest* 34 (January 1928): 2.

64. Ibid., 5.

65. Ibid.

66. Ibid., 7.

67. Southard, the mother of dental assisting, managed to seal her reputation as a dental assistant of unquestionable loyalty and devotion to the profession by dying of a heart attack while attending a banquet of the Florida Dental Assistants' Association on November 12, 1940. The ADAA commemorated her birthday for many years thereafter. "A Gallant Little Lady Passes On," *The Dental Assistant* 10 (January-February 1941): 3.

68. Neville S. Hoff, "How Shall the Profession Meet Its New Obligations Resulting from Its Propaganda for Popular Education in Oral Hygiene and Preventive Dentistry?" as published by *The Dental Cosmos* 54 (July 1912): 784.

69. Ibid.

70. Grace P. Rogers, "The Graduate Dentist Versus the Dental Nurse," *Dentist's Magazine* 1 (June 1906): 649.

71. Ibid.

72. Thomas Barrett, "A New Species of Dentist: Do We Want It?" as published by *The Dental Cosmos* 61 (December 1919): 1207, and H. J. Burkhart, cited by Harry Beck in his letter to the editor of *The Dental Cosmos* 62 [March 1920]: 387, respectively.

73. Raymond Albray, "Do We Need a Dental Nurse or Something to Talk About?" *New Jersey Dental Journal* 1 (September 1912): 274–275.

74. Barrett, "A New Species of Dentist: Do We Want It?" 1207.

75. Beck to the editor of *The Dental Cosmos* 62: 387.

76. Dental assistants did so in 1924; hygienists, in 1923.

77. George Wood Clapp, "The Rise and Fall of Oral Hygiene in Bridgeport (Second Article)," *Dental Digest* 34 (February 1928): 91

78. George Wood Clapp, "The Rise and Fall of Oral Hygiene in Bridgeport (Third Article)," *Dental Digest* 34 (March 1928): 172

79. George Wood Clapp, "The Rise and Fall of Oral Hygiene in Bridgeport (Fourth Article)," *Dental Digest* 34 (April 1928): 252–253.

80. Hart, "Working Out the Details," 1129

81. Ibid., 1130.

82. Ibid., 1130.

83. Rose House, "Work of the Preventive Dental Clinic in the Bridgeport Public Schools," as published by *The Dental Cosmos* 57 (October 1915): 1133. There was no indication of whether the teachers had volunteered, or the school principal had commandeered, the room for this use.

84. For "missionaries to the home," see Clapp, "Rise and Fall (Fourth Article)," 258. For "the Gospel of clean mouths," see Hart, "Working Out the Details,"1131.

85. Hart, "Working Out the Details," 1130–1131.

86. Clapp, "The Rise and Fall (Fourth Article)," 258.

87. House, "Work of the Preventive Dental Clinic," 1135.

88. Ibid., 1136. The New York City children serviced by the Children's Aid Society clinic, "whose parents are too poor to send them to the public schools," were similarly appreciative. One "was a small, bright-looking boy, who pleaded so hard to be taken in that he was told that if he would wait until all the other children in attendance that day had been cared for . . . he might receive treatment. This boy lived in the Bronx and traveled nearly ten miles each way in coming to the clinic." Arthur H. Merritt, "The Dental Clinics of the Children's Aid Society," *Oral Hygiene* 1 (December 1911): 911–918. (914)

89. Clapp, "The Rise and Fall (Fourth Article)," 258.

90. Hart, "Working Out the Details," 1130.

91. Ibid., 1131–1132.

92. George Wood Clapp, "The Rise and Fall of Oral Hygiene in Bridgeport (Fifth Article)," *Dental Digest* 34 (May 1928): 320–321

93. Ibid., 322.

94. George Wood Clapp, "The Rise and Fall of Oral Hygiene in Bridgeport (Eleventh Article)," *Dental Digest* 34 (November 1928): 781.

95. Richard Grady, "Cooperation of the Public Schools in Teaching 'Good Teeth, Good Health,'" as published by *American Journal of Dental Science* 35 (August 1904): 141.

96. Luther Gulick, "Why 250,000 Children Quit School," *Oral Hygiene* 1 (January 1911): 20, 22.

97. M. Evangeline Jordan, "Teeth and Taxes," *Dental Digest* 20 (February 1914): 114.

98. Otto King, "Oral Hygiene and Its Relation to Public and Individual Health," as published by the *Journal of the National Dental Association* 4 (February 1917): 149.

99. H. C. Brown, "Attitude of the State Government toward Public Health," as published by *The Dental Brief* 15 (July 1910): 575.

100. Other examples of stories directed at children included George Cunningham's lecture, "My Hobby," in which he proposed that members of his child audience consider making a hobby of dental care. "One good thing about making a hobby of your teeth," he said, "is you always carry your collection about with you" (George Cunningham, "My Hobby," *Oral Hygiene* 4 [December 1912]: 1036). The production of materials in this genre extended over an extremely long interval; see, for example, not only the playlets listed here, but the stories "The Cave People" and "The Twins" (the latter about central incisors), published in 1932, and the playlet "Grandfather Molar," of the same year. (Elma Miller, "The Cave People," *Dental Digest* 38 (February 1932): 71–72; "The Twins," *Dental Digest* 38 (March 1932): pages unknown; and Lon Morrey, "Grandfather Molar: A Dental Health Playlet," *Dental Digest* 38 (July 1932): 244–249.)

101. Evelyn Wright Nelson, "Mouth Hygiene: A Health Symposium Playlet for Young People," *Oral Hygiene* 3 no. 12, (December 1913): 969.

102. Ibid., 970.

103. Ibid., 970.

104. Ibid., 973

105. Ibid.

106. Ibid., 968.

107. Ibid.

108. Ibid., 971.

109. "Good Teeth for School Children," as reprinted in *The Dental Brief* 16 (March 1911): 219.

110. Charles Wolff, "Dentistry for the Rich and the Poor," *Dental Digest* 26 (March 1920): 139.

Chapter 2 — Diet and the Dental Critique of American Life

1. As Diane Paul argues, "In the United States, Canada, Britain, and much of Europe, the concept of genetic perfectibility underlay some of the most sharply defined fissures in the intellectual and moral landscape. . . . We now know that eugenics

was a more diverse movement, enjoying much broader political support, than one would imagine from conventional accounts" (Diane Paul, *Controlling Human Heredity: 1865 to the Present* [Atlantic Highlands, NJ: Humanities Press, 1995]: 2, 19). For more on the scientists who were involved in the study of human heredity, and on the political, cultural, and health-care manifestations of this interest, see also Daniel J. Kevles, *In the Name of Eugenics: Genetics and the Uses of Human Heredity* (Cambridge, MA: Harvard University Press, 1985), Alan M. Kraut, *Silent Travelers: Germs, Genes, and the "Immigrant Menace"* (Baltimore: Johns Hopkins University Press, 1994), and Martin S. Pernick, *The Black Stork: Eugenics and the Death of "Defective" Babies in American Medicine and Motion Pictures Since 1915* (New York: Oxford University Press, 1996).

2. Eugene Talbot, "Dental and Facial Evidences of Constitutional Defect," as published in *The International Dental Journal* 17 (May 1896): 269.

3. Ibid., 263.

4. Eugene Talbot, "Laws Governing Eugenesis: A Thirty-five Years' Study of Developmental Pathology," *The Dental Era* 4 (June 1905): 298.

5. Eugene Talbot, "Stigmata of Degeneracy in Relation to Irregularities of the Teeth," as published by *Dental Review* 16 (March 15, 1902): 192.

6. Eugene Talbot, "The Degenerate Jaws and Teeth," as published by *The International Dental Journal* 18 (February 1897): 80.

7. Eugene Talbot, "Anatomic Changes in the Head, Face, Jaws, and Teeth in the Evolution of Man," as published by *Dental Digest* 10 (December 1904): 1422.

8. Talbot, "Stigmata of Degeneracy in Relation to Irregularities of the Teeth," 192.

9. Talbot, "Anatomic Changes in the Head, Face, Jaws, and Teeth," 1430. At other times, Talbot added "hysterics, liars, pessimists, and sentimentalists" to the list. See, for example, Talbot, "Stigmata of Degeneracy in Relation to Irregularities of the Teeth," 191.

10. O. A. Weiss comments on Talbot, "Stigmata of Degeneracy in Relation to Irregularities of the Teeth," 219.

11. Eugene Talbot, "Constitutional Causes of Tooth Decay," as published by *Dental Digest* 9 (December 1903): 1436.

12. Eugene Talbot, "Developmental Pathology and Tooth Decay," as published by *The Dental Cosmos* 47 (December 1905): 1436.

13. Talbot, "Laws Governing Eugenesis," 299.

14. Talbot, "The Degenerate Jaws and Teeth," 76.

15. Eugene Talbot, "My Fifty-three Years of Professional Life," *The Pacific Dental Gazette* 30 (July 1922): 391.

16. Talbot, "Anatomic Changes in the Head, Face, Jaws, and Teeth," 1424. "Ordinary" consanguineous marriage, Talbot believed, could be practiced without impunity if one were confident that one's genetic inheritance was absolutely sound: otherwise he considered it wiser to seek a mate outside of one's own family tree. "Socially" consanguineous marriages, in which partners had been "living under similar conditions, habits, and surroundings, laboring at the same occupation, [and] indulging in the same dissipation . . . [which] tend to engender like diseases and degenerations irrespective of any blood relationship," could be just as unwise as "ordinary" consanguineous marriages, and Talbot advised against them. "[Social consanguinity] has largely aided real or family consanguinity in the production of the diseases and degenerations which have so heavily fallen

upon the aristocracies and royal families of Europe." (Eugene Talbot, "Social Consanguinity, Near Kin, Early and Late Marriage," *International Dental Journal* 22 [May 1901]: 299.)

17. Talbot, "Anatomic Changes, in the Head, Face, Jaws, and Teeth," 1426.

18. Hect Boethius quoted by Burton (*Anatomy of Melancholy*, 1652), as cited by Talbot, "Anatomic Changes in the Head, Face, Jaws, and Teeth," 1425.

19. "Dr. Channing," comments on Talbot, "Social Consanguinity, Near Kin, Early and Late Marriage," 449.

20. Ibid., 451.

21. Ibid., 450.

22. F. G. Corey, "Physical Conditions," *Western Dental Journal* 20 (December 1906): 836.

23. F. G. Corey, " 'Making Good,' (The Physical Conditions of the Teeth)," as published by *Western Dental Journal* 20 (August 1906): 536.

24. Ibid., 535.

25. Ibid., 535.

26. Ibid., 539.

27. C. A. Martin, comments on F. G. Corey, "'Making Good,'" 540. The dentist ceded absolutely no ground on the issue of miscegenation, though: "For myself," he concluded, "I think there are plenty of physically perfect people of my own race and color to take car [sic] of my posterity, and I do not care to have my blood mixed up with a little off-color."

28. As Laura Shapiro has observed of a weekly menu devised by such zealots, "To balance a meal by numbers alone, ignoring taste and texture, meant that creamed potatoes, creamed vegetable soup, macaroni with cream sauce, salad with a creamy dressing, and gelatin with cream were all listed on the menu [on the same day]." Mathematical thinking about food—together with an acknowledgment of Americans' world-renowned taste for sweets—also led the Boston Cooking School Magazine to recommend frosting sandwiches for children's lunchboxes in 1898. Laura Shapiro, *Perfection Salad: Women and Cooking at the Turn of the Century* (New York: Farrar, Straus, Giroux, 1986): 209, 211.

29. Harvey Levenstein, *Revolution at the Table: The Transformation of the American Diet* (New York: Oxford University Press, 1988): 31.

30. Harvey Levenstein, *Paradox of Plenty: A Social History of Eating in Modern America* (New York: Oxford University Press, 1993): 27.

31. Levenstein, *Revolution at the Table*, 87. Widely acclaimed for his physical stamina (in 1902, "the five-foot-six Fletcher had climbed the 854 steps of the Washington Monument and then bounded down them without resting"), Fletcher won the attention of many prominent Americans, including the Army Chief of Staff and the eminent Yale professor of physiology Russell Chittenden, to whom Fletcher sent his odorless stools through the US mail (evidence, he alleged, of the particularly complete digestion begun by thorough chewing). Ibid., 88.

32. As cited in Shapiro, *Perfection Salad*, 213.

33. See, for example, Regina Kunzel, *Fallen Women, Problem Girls: Unmarried Mothers and the Professionalization of Social Work, 1890–1945* (New Haven: Yale University Press, 1993).

34. "A prime objective," Levenstein writes of the social workers' approach to Mexican Americans, "was to convince them to abandon the traditional Mexican sauces (whose tomatoes and chiles provided vitamins and whose nuts and cheese pro-

vided protein, calcium, and vitamins) in favor of only two sauces: White Sauce, consisting of flour, butter and milk, and Hard Sauce, mainly sugar and butter." Levenstein, *Revolution at the Table*, 157.

35. This was at least partly because of the centrality of food to Italian Americans' ethnic identity, and partly due to nutritionists' promotion of pasta as an economical source of protein during the Depression. On the resistance to assimilation of Italians, see Hasia R. Diner, *Hungering for America: Italian, Irish, and Jewish Foodways in the Age of Migration* (Cambridge: Harvard University Press, 2001), especially the comment of Saul Alinsky that "these Welfare workers would get upset because poor Italian families insisted on buying very good olive oil to cook with . . . Italians have to have olive oil . . . it's something much more important than budgets or stuff like that" (56). Nevertheless, as Harvey Levenstein points out, "The versions [of Italian foods] served were very much adapted to American tastes. Rarely did recipes for tomato-based sauces call for even a scrap of the dreaded garlic clove. *Good Housekeeping*'s recipe for spaghetti and meatballs called for beef suet, horseradish, and 'bottled condiment sauce' in the meatballs, but no garlic in the accompanying tomato sauce. . . . For its version of that dish, *American Cookery* had cooks flavor two cans of tomato soup with a tablespoon of Worcestershire sauce. . . . Some people . . . even used ketchup as the tomato sauce, as did the US Army" (Levenstein, *Paradox of Plenty*, 30).

36. On infant feeding and its relationship to infant mortality, see Richard Meckel, *Save the Babies: American Public Health Reform and the Prevention of Infant Mortality, 1850–1929* (Baltimore: Johns Hopkins University Press, 1990), especially chapter 3, "Pure Milk for Babies: Improving the Urban Milk Supply."

37. Mellin's Food even advertised to physicians its "NEW labels . . . NO directions" in a 1932 volume of the Journal of the American Medical Association. Rima Apple, *Mothers and Medicine: A Social History of Infant Feeding, 1890–1940* (Madison: University of Wisconsin Press, 1987): 91.

38. Ibid., 107.

39. Rima Apple, *Vitamania: Vitamins in American Culture* (New Brunswick, NJ: Rutgers University Press, 1996): 6.

40. T. E. Powell, comments on A. B. Spach's "Diet in Health and Disease," as published by *Dental Review* 19 (June 15, 1905): 564.

41. B. J. Cigrand, comments on Spach's "Diet in Health and Disease," 571.

42. On public health officials and food regulation, see Meckel, *Save the Babies*, 67.

43. B. J. Cigrand, "Diet, Dentures and Disposition," *Dental Review* 18 (February 15, 1904): 147.

44. Alfred W. McCann, "Agriculture or Human Culture—Which?" as republished by *Dental Digest* 25 (August 1919): 505. (Originally published in the *New York Globe*, no date given.)

45. M. Evangeline Jordon, "Feeding the Child from the Standpoint of a Dentist," as published by the *Journal of the American Dental Association 10* (August 1923): 743.

46. Guy A. Woods, discussion of Jordon, "Feeding the Child," 748.

47. W. H. Card, discussion of Jordon, "Feeding the Child," 749.

48. Paul A. Barker, discussion of Jordon, "Feeding the Child," 749.

49. (Author's name withheld), "A Dentist's Wife and His Health," *Dental Digest* 28 (November 1922): 741–743.

50. "Educating the Public," *Dental Digest* 28 (November 1922): 740.

51. C. Frank Bliven, comments on H. D. Perky's paper "Nutrition as a Tooth-Builder," as published by *The Dental Cosmos* 43 (June 1901): 671.

52. Gustave Wiksell, "Hammer and Nails," as published by *The Dental Cosmos* 44 (August 1902): 869.

53. C. P. Webster, "One Cause of Dental Degeneration: The Physical Relation of Food to the Teeth," *The Dental Cosmos* 40 (February 1898): 139.

54. H. T. Harvey, "Toothless Twentieth Centenarians; or, Vegetarianism, Which?" *Ohio Dental Journal* 19 (February 1899): 119.

55. Cigrand, "Diet, Dentures and Disposition," 108.

56. H. D. Perky, "Nutrition as a Tooth-Builder," as published by *The Dental Cosmos* 43 (June 1901): 671.

57. "A Chemist's Adventure in 'Jam,'" *Dental Digest* 28 (May 1922): 340.

58. Spach, "Diet in Health and Disease," 529.

59. "We Must Win!" *Dental Digest* 24 (June 1918): 449. The failure to capitalize the initial "g" in "german" was intended as an intentional snub.

60. Wiksell, "Hammer and Nails," 869.

61. C. Frank Bliven, comments on Perky, "Nutrition as a Tooth-Builder," 671.

62. Wiksell, "Hammer and Nails," 870.

63. "Dr. Barrett," comments on Wiksell, "Hammer and Nails," 872. Barrett pointed out, with some disdain, that a late member of the Northeastern Dental Society had made a similar presentation on the evils of refined flour at every meeting of the organization.

64. Ibid., 871. Complaints about dietary faddism recurred frequently, sometimes inspiring harsh words at dental society meetings. In 1905, one dentist decried the "raw food mania," saying that "Some freak like Dowie or Mrs. Eddy had a dream that raw food is the thing and nature's only way, tried it upon himself and thought he found it good, and induced others to do the same" (Spach, "Diet in Health and Disease," 527). In response, another dentist demanded to know "what relation Mrs Eddy bears to the subject-matter of the paper," and whether Spach had ever actually read Mary Baker Eddy's magnum opus, "Science and Health." ("(These questions were not answered)," the editors reported.) (C. F. Hart, comments on Spach, "Diet in Health and Disease," 570.)

65. Albert B. King, "Bakers' Bread as a Factor in Inducing Dental Caries," as published by *The Dental Cosmos* 55 (May 1913): 510.

66. Cigrand, "Diet, Dentures, and Disposition," 102. Another writer described his hope that a change in the American diet would cause Americans to "lose our reputation abroad as being people who are suffering from dyspepsia, or the 'Yankee disease'": it is not entirely clear whether it was the dyspepsia or the decay itself that was known as the "Yankee disease" (Ibid. 138). Arthur D. Black, son of the legendary Illinois dentist Greene Vardiman Black (who had innovated new methods of preparing cavities for filling, and who invented the foot-treadle dental drill), disputed Cigrand's claim that dyspepsia could cause tooth decay: "I do not believe that eructations of acids into the mouth, no matter how frequently, would be a primary cause of caries of the teeth," Black argued. He endorsed H. T. Harvey's earlier and less direct connection between dyspepsia, a poor constitution, and dental decay: "Caries of the teeth in such cases occurs more particularly from the general condition of the body, making the person more susceptible to the disease" (Arthur D. Black, comments on Cigrand, 146).

67. "Candy on the Grill: Enquiry by Dr. H. G. Harvitt Decries Candy-Eating as Dangerous," *Dental Digest* 28 (April 1922): 273–274. The *Digest* described Harvitt's survey, which was mailed to twenty American dentists, as "unbiased in its wording, covering these two questions: 1. What does your experience show to be the effect of excessive candy-eating on teeth not cared for regularly? 2. What can you suggest to offset the evil inherent in the situation?" Two specialists nevertheless found room to express their opinion that "candy is an important element of the diet and is conducive to general and dental health," a fact which the *Digest* editors reported without comment other than its placement in the midst of an otherwise resounding verbal trouncing of the candy habit. (Ibid, 274).

68. Jordon, "Feeding the Child," 746.

69. Anna De Planter, "Nutrition: Its Relation to Mouth Hygiene," as published by *The Dental Cosmos* 65 (November 1923): 1177.

70. Lou Lombard, "Spare the Sweets and Save the Teeth," *Journal of the American Dental Association* 11 (December 1924): 1246–1247. Public schools' practice of permitting the sale of candy—in some cases, it seems, the school doing the selling itself—seemed to Lombard to require explanation. Then as now, the need to raise money for the school was the chief justification for the practice: Lombard listed "playground apparatus; victrola; money for graduation; milk for children who cannot afford to buy it; tables and chairs for use in the lower grades; a trip to Washington; a medicine cabinet" as among the schools' needs. "These may all be very desirable and necessary, but is there no other way to get them?" he asked. (Ibid, 1248.) Modern schools have been every bit as unsuccessful in finding "some other way to get" such items: for more on public schools' collaboration with producers of junk food in the 1990s, see Marion Nestle, *Food Politics: How the Food Industry Influences Nutrition and Health* (Berkeley: University of California Press, 2002), especially chapter 9, "Pushing Soft Drinks," in which Nestle describes the "pouring rights" contracts that major soft drink producers have negotiated with American school districts.

71. Harvey, "Toothless Twentieth Centenarians," 120–121.

72. J. F. Teufert, "Diet," *Oral Hygiene* 1 (September 1911): 655.

73. Editor's introduction to Teufert, "Diet," 654.

74. G. A. Ostermeier, "One Swallow Made an Eternity," *Oral Hygiene* 1 (September 1911): 666.

75. Spach, "Diet in Health and Disease," 526.

76. Ibid., 527.

77. Charles Cochrane, "The Crime of Uneducated Eating," *Western Dental Journal* 21 [orig. *Metropolitan Magazine*] (October 1907): 738. Dentists also considered farmers' "habits of eating" off-limits to dentists themselves: "The dentist should take a light lunch, and, in my judgment, a comparatively light breakfast; but he is free to take the greater part of his food at the evening meal, when he is supposed to have his evening free from the more strenuous activities of mind and body," argued Frederick Noyes in 1905. "They need something, but they do not need a heavy meal at noon, because they must go back to the acute concentration of mind necessary for the rapid execution of detailed performance, which is impossible without a strong supply of blood in the central nervous system" (Frederick B. Noyes, comments on Spach, "Diet in Health and Disease," 567–568).

78. C. P. Pruyn, comments on Cigrand, "Diet, Dentures and Disposition," 143.

79. "Prof. Sedgwick," "The Real American Peril," *Dental Digest* 24 (July 1918): 448–449.

80. J. P. Buckley, "Address of the President of the American Dental Association," as published by the *Journal of the American Dental Association* 10 (November 1923): 994.

81. S. C. Sims, "The Importance of Diet in the Maintenance of a Healthy Condition of the Oral Cavity," as published by *Dental Review* 19 (January 15, 1905): 18

82. Clarence H. Wright, comments on Spach, "Diet in Health and Disease," 571.

83. Ibid., 571.

84. "A Member of the Rochester Dental Society," "The Story of Tim (Continued from January Issue)," *Dental Digest* 17 (February 1911): 116.

85. Ibid., 116.

86. McCann, "Agriculture or Human Culture—Which?" 506.

87. "The Story of Tim," 116.

88. On Darwin's and Galton's views, see Paul, *Controlling Human Heredity*, especially chapter 2, "Evolutionary Anxieties."

89. Harvey, "Toothless Twentieth Centenarians," 120.

90. Frederick B. Noyes, comments on Spach's "Diet in Health and Disease," 566.

91. Teufert, "Diet," 655.

92. Sim Wallace, "Why Our Civilization Has Given Us Poor Teeth," *American Dental Journal* 10 (January 15, 1913): 328.

93. Ibid., 328, 330.

94. "Raw Carrots as an Important Factor in Dental Hygiene," *The Dental Cosmos* 55 (February 1913): 208.

95. Buckley, "Address of the President," 995.

96. Jordon, "Feeding the Child," 743.

97. L. O. Frech, comments on Lydia Roberts, "Better Nutrition of Children," as published by the *Journal of the American Dental Association* 10 (December 23): 1134.

98. Clara Davis, "A Report on the Self-Selection Diet Experiment in Infants and Young Children," *Journal of the American Dental Association* 18 (June 1931): 1144.

99. Ibid., 1148, 1151–1152. On weight gain as a measure of infant and child health, see Jeffrey P. Brosco, "Weight Charts and Well Child Care: When the Pediatrician Became the Expert in Child Health," in Stern and Markel, *Formative Years,* 91–120.

100. Davis, "Report on the Self-Selection Diet Experiment," 1153.

101. Claude C. Chick, "Thoughtless Mothers," *American Journal of Dental Science* 32 (March 1899): 524.

102. "The Story of Tim," 52.

103. Alfred Fones, "Prenatal Diet and Its Relation to the Teeth," as published in the *Journal of the American Dental Association* 10 (November 1923): 1029

104. Weston Price, "Our Children: How We May Add to or Subtract from Their Inheritance," unpublished lecture, circa 1929, pages 7, 18. Price-Pottenger Foundation Archive, La Mesa, CA. This and all materials from the PPNF archive used with kind permission of The Price-Pottenger Nutrition Foundation™ Board of Directors, www.ppnf.org.

105. Weston Price, *Nutrition and Physical Degeneration* (New York: Paul B. Hoeber, Inc., 1935): 127.

106. Ibid., 116.

107. Weston Price, "Manual for Lecture #2, Descriptive Text for Numbered Illustra-tions, Lecture Series Reporting Light from Primitive Races on Modern Degenera-tion" (Cleveland: Dental Research Laboratories [self-published], no date available): 12.

108. Weston Price, "Why Dental Caries with Modern Civilizations? Field Studies among the Polynesians and Melanesians of the South Sea Islands," *Dental Digest*, May 1935: 164.

109. Price, *Nutrition and Physical Degeneration*, 193.

110. Ibid., 193.

111. Letter of Norman Price, MD, to Weston Price, July 11, 1939, File: "Price Correspon-dence," Price-Pottenger Foundation Archive, La Mesa, CA.

112. Ibid.

113. Price, *Nutrition and Physical Degeneration*, 211.

114. Price, "Why Dental Caries with Modern Civilizations?" 193.

115. More recently, renewed interest in the deficiencies of the American diet, and Michael Pollan's book *The Omnivore's Dilemma*, which mentions Price's work, have facilitated a small boom in Price-related scholarship and advocacy. Pollan, *The Omnivore's Dilemma* (New York: Penguin, 2006).

Chapter 3 — "Like a Sugar-Coated Pill"

1. "A Japanese Office Boy Writes," *Dental Digest* 27 (March 1921): 194–185.

2. Ibid., 194.

3. Dental travel writing thus reflected the characteristics that literary critic Mary Louise Pratt has identified in travel writing more broadly: "While the imperial metropolis tends to understand itself as determining the periphery (in the ema-nating glow of the civilizing mission or the cash flow of development, for exam-ple), it habitually blinds itself to the ways in which the periphery determines the metropolis—beginning, perhaps, with the latter's obsessive need to present and re-present its peripheries and its others continually to itself. Travel writing, among other institutions, is heavily organized in the service of that imperative." Mary Louise Pratt, *Imperial Eyes: Travel Writing and Transculturation* (New York: Routledge, 1992): 6.

4. In this respect, they served a function similar to that of medical journals. See Kenneth Ludmerer, *Learning to Heal: The Development of American Medical Edu-cation* (Baltimore: Johns Hopkins University Press, 1985): 87.

5. D. T. Parkinson, "Dentistry Around the World," *Oral Hygiene* 17 (March 1927): 444. Parkinson was the lone dentist in the tour group, comprised of 450 under-graduates (including 50 "girls and young women").

6. I have followed modern practices in the spelling of place names which were often Anglicized (e.g., "Hawaii" and "Porto Rico") by contemporaries, but have left con-temporary usages intact when I have excerpted them directly.

7. H. J. La Salle, "Dental Conditions in Samoa," *Northwest Journal of Dentistry* 21 (July 1933): 17.

8. S. D. Boak, "Some Observations during Three Years' Service in the Tropics," *Den-tal Summary* 27 (May 1907): 330.

9. "Winning Souls Through the Dental Forceps," *Dental Digest* 27 (April 1921): 229–230.

10. Ibid., 230.

11. "From Far India," *Dental Summary* 41 (September 1921): 810.

12. "Wanted, Dentists in Persia," *The Dental Cosmos* 63 (November 1921): 1150.

13. "Chinese Dentists Use Unique Methods," *Oral Hygiene* 10 (June 1920): 854.

14. Walther Buchler, "Dentistry in India," *Dental Digest* 37 (March 1931): 170.

15. "Dentistry in Hongkong," *Western Dental Journal* 30 (May 1916): 49.

16. Boak, "Some Observations during Three Years' Service in the Tropics," 257.

17. James H. Howell, "Dentistry in Northern Russia," *Bulletin of the Michigan State Dental Society* 1 (March 1919): 6.

18. George Cecil, "The Kaffir Dentist," *The Dental Brief* 8, no. 9 (September 1903): 528.

19. "A Returned Soldier," "Filipino Dentistry," *The Dental Brief* 7, no. 1 (January 1902): 76.

20. "Medical and Dental Practice in China," *The Dental Brief* 8, no. 1, (January 1903): 32.

21. Weston Price, *Nutrition and Physical Degeneration* (New York: Paul B. Hoeber, Inc., 1935): 118.

22. Cecil, "The Kaffir Dentist," 528.

23. George Cecil, "India: The Native Dentist," *The Dental Brief* 7, no. 12 (December 1902): 694.

24. George Cecil, "Dentistry in Gibraltar and Malta," *The Dental Brief* 9, no. 6 (June 1904): 355.

25. "A Returned Soldier," "Filipino Dentistry," 77.

26. Cecil, "The Kaffir Dentist," 529.

27. George Cecil, "Dentistry in China," *Dental Digest* 28, no. 8 (August 1922): 515.

28. George Cecil, "Dental Surgery in India: An Awful Experience," *The Dental Brief* 8, no. 12 (December 1903): 711.

29. Cecil traveled widely, and spent time in several countries where the Spanish word "siesta" would have been used to describe a midday nap. It would not have been used by either Englishmen or Indians in this time period, however, so Cecil's insistence on it here suggests again his tendency to link brownness with disrespect for time—and to homogenize brownness itself quite dramatically.

30. Ibid., 712.

31. George Cecil, "The European Dentist in India and the Prospects Awaiting Him," *The Dental Brief* 7 (October 1902): 548.

32. Cecil, "The Kaffir Dentist," 529.

33. Cecil, "Dentistry in Gibraltar and Malta," 355.

34. Cecil, "The Kaffir Dentist," 528.

35. Ibid.

36. The ideas that "savages" were generally less susceptible to pain than were the "civilized" had its origins in nineteenth-century medicine: see, for example, Martin Pernick, *A Calculus of Suffering: Pain, Professionalism, and Anesthesia in Nineteenth-Century America* (New York: Columbia University Press, 1985), especially chapter 7, "They Don't Feel It Like We Do: Social Politics and the Perception of Pain." Alcohol use was widely understood to exert an anesthetic effect, though greater sensitivity to pain was said to prevail among habitual inebriates deprived of alcohol. By either theory, the "Kaffir" would have been entitled to less sympathy from his dentist, and from Cecil.

37. Cecil, "The European Dentist in India," 543.
38. Ibid., 544.
39. Ibid., 548.
40. Landis Wirt, "Observations of an American Dentist in India," *Dental Digest* 17, no. 10 (October 1911): 621.
41. George Cecil, "Dentistry in the British Army," *The Dental Brief* 19, no. 11 (November 1913): 625.
42. Ibid., 628.
43. George Cecil, "European Dentists in India," *Oral Hygiene* 18, no. 9 (September 1928): 1692.
44. Cecil, "The European Dentist in India," 549.
45. George Cecil, "Concerning Dentists in India," *The Dental Brief* 8 (January 1903): 8.
46. Albert Nahas, "A Plea on Behalf of American Dentistry," *The Dental Cosmos* 61, no. 3 (March 1919): 222.
47. "Chinese Dentists' Dark Ways," *Dental Digest* 25 (November 1919): 675.
48. N. S. Jenkins, "The Influence of American Dentists upon Europe," *The Dental Cosmos* 59 (February 1917): 179.
49. Ibid., 184.
50. "The Japanese Situation," *Military Dental Journal* 6 (December 1923): 216.
51. Transcribed address of E. C. Kirk in the "Proceedings of the Connecticut Dental Hygiene Association Fifth Annual Meeting, Bridgeport, CT, May 23–24 1919," *The Dental Cosmos* 62 (May 1920): 657.
52. Some historians place the Filipino death toll as high as one million, including war-related civilian deaths due to illness, injury, and displacement. See Matthew Frye Jacobson, "Imperial Amnesia: Teddy Roosevelt, the Philippines, and the Modern Art of Forgetting," *Radical History Review* 73 (1999): 119.
53. "A Returned Soldier," "Filipino Dentistry," 73.
54. Ibid., figures p. 75, 77.
55. "Barbarism" was one step above "savagery" in the hierarchy imagined by US imperialists. Louis Ottofy, "The Teeth of the Igorots," *The Dental Cosmos* 50 (July 1908): 687.
56. "A Regular," "Teeth of the Head Hunters of Mindanao—Fantastic Designs and Grewsome Effects," *Dental Review* 18 (April 15, 1904): 319.
57. Ibid., 324.
58. Louis Ottofy, "History of Dentistry in the Philippine Islands," *The Dental Cosmos* 57 (September 1905): 1098.
59. Ibid., 1100.
60. For more on the role of the Igorots in the St. Louis Exposition, see Paul Kramer, "Making Concessions: Race and Empire Revisited at the Philippine Exposition, St. Louis, 1901–1905," *Radical History Review* 73 (1999): 74–114.
61. Ottofy, "Teeth of the Igorots," 670–671. On the World's Fair participants' unwilling repatriation to the Philippines, see Kramer, "Making Concessions," especially page 106. After the St. Louis Exposition, a group of Igorot and Moros expressed, through a translator, their interest in remaining to tour the United States in exchange for Exposition wages and three hours of school per day. World's Fair officials rejected this suggestion, and tricked the group into boarding a train to Seattle "under the guise of an outing" to the Midway at the fair.

62. Ottofy, "Teeth of the Igorots," 684.

63. Ottofy reported that "It was almost impossible to secure the girls, who would run and scream and hide." Ibid., 674–675.

64. Ibid., 694.

65. Ibid.

66. Ibid.

67. Ibid.

68. On the origins of military governors as "Indian fighters," see Federico Magdalena, "Moro-American Relations in the Philippines," *Philippine Studies* 44 (Third Quarter, 1996): 430. Ottofy's commitment to the propagation of American dental standards continued after his return to the United States in 1920, when he co-founded the International College of Dentists, an organization that sought to "study the progress of the dental profession and distribute the information to all countries of the world." International health and government officials were invited to nominate for membership in the college "the ablest, most progressive, best educated, ethical practitioner in [each] country, regardless of his place of domicile, nationality, race, color or religion." As the College reported, "the request was so faithfully carried out that in many instances no nomination could be made on the grounds that, 'There is no dentist practicing in the country who can be recommended in accordance with the high ideals of the College.'" http://www.icd.org/history.htm, accessed May 24, 2008.

69. See, for example, Boak, "Some Observations during Three Years' Service," 260–268, especially his tale of a removable gold dental decoration being shared among family members in Tarlac.

70. Ibid., 264.

71. Ibid.

72. Ibid.

73. Lewis Maly, "Dentistry in Morodom," *Military Dental Journal* 5 (September 1922): 140.

74. Magdalena, "Moro-American Relations in the Philippines," 437. Magdalena argues that the Moros actually objected to Americans' withdrawal from the Philippines (as, he claims, did Christian Filipinos in Moro territory), and locates in the Moros' resistance to Christian Filipino rule the origins of what he calls "the Wild, Wild West in Mindanao" today. What was once known as Moroland is now the seat of the Islamic fundamentalist Abu Sayyaf rebel movement.

75. The dominant "sugar factors" were the five large corporations engaged in the fractioning of Hawai'ian sugar cane into its factorial parts—molasses and a variety of purified cane sugars. John Whitehead writes that by the 1930s, these five corporations controlled "96 percent of Hawai'i's sugar crop as well as a substantial portion of the pineapple industry. They dominated shipping to and from the islands through the Matson Line, and they also controlled the major wholesale and retail mercantile functions in the islands. In addition to their dominance of the economic sphere, the Big Five exerted substantial political influence in territorial Hawai'i through the Republican Party, which dominated the territorial legislature prior to World War II. Many of the appointed territorial governors had a connection to the Big Five firms as officers or investors." John S. Whitehead, "Western Progressives, Old South Planters, or Colonial Oppressors: The Enigma of Hawai'i's 'Big Five,' 1898–1940," *Western Historical Quarterly* 30 (Autumn 1999): 297.

76. F. H. Metcalf, "Honolulu as I Found It," *Pacific Dental Gazette* 17 (January 1901): 20.

77. Ibid., 21.

78. Martha R. Jones, Nils P. Larsen, and George P. Pritchard, "Dental Disease in Hawaii—Odontoclasia: A Clinically Significant Unrecognized Form of Tooth Decay in the Pre-School Child of Honolulu," *The Dental Cosmos* 72 (May 1930): 439.

79. Helen Baukin, "Kapaa School, Kauai, Hawaiian Islands," *Journal of the American Dental Association* 17 (February 1930): 360.

80. Ibid., 361.

81. Ibid., 362.

82. *Hawaii Educational Review* 12 (1923): 21, as cited in B. K. Hyams, "School Teachers as Agents of Cultural Imperialism in Territorial Hawai'i," *Journal of Pacific History* 20 (October 1985): 217.

83. Ibid., 205.

84. Ibid., 362. Hawai'i was neither a sovereign nation nor a state in this period, but Baukin apparently regarded its status as a US territory as temporary: hence her belief that the United States was, for purposes of patriotic displays, the "country" of Hawai'ian schoolchildren.

85. H. Dorothy Dudley, "Dental Practice in Hawaii," *Journal of the Michigan State Dental Society* 18 (April 1936): 95. For more on the expropriation of Hawai'ian culture, and particularly Hawai'ian music and dance, see Elizabeth Buck, *Paradise Remade: The Politics of Culture and History in Hawai'i* (Philadelphia: Temple University Press, 1993).

86. Dudley, "Dental Practice in Hawaii," 95.

87. "Bureau of Public Relations: Dental Health Education and Service for the Children in Hawaii," *Journal of the American Dental Association* 25/The *Dental Cosmos* 80 (November 1938): 1864–1867. The *Journal of the American Dental Association* and *The Dental Cosmos*, the two most venerable of American dental magazines, merged in 1937. Volume numbering and pagination, as I have used them here, continued in series with past issues of the *Journal of the American Dental Association*, though 1938 issues included both sets of volume and page numbers.

88. James Voigt, "Dentistry in Hawaii," *Dental Students' Magazine* 43 (November 1964): 119–121.

Chapter 4 — "This National Stupidity"

1. Frank W. Rounds, "Democracy at the Crossroads," *New England Dental Journal* 2 (April 1949): 14–15.

2. On American programs of social insurance, see Theda Skocpol, *Protecting Soldiers and Mothers: The Political Origins of Social Policy in the United States* (Cambridge: Harvard University Press, 1992). On physicians' responses to such programs, see Paul Starr, *The Social Transformation of American Medicine: The Rise of a Sovereign Profession and the Making of a Vast Industry* (New York: Basic Books, 1982).

3. In Roman Catholic iconology, St. Apollonia is the patroness of those with toothache. Frederick A. Keyes, "Dental Philanthropy; Its Uses and Abuses," *Oral Hygiene* 4 (February 1914): 104–105.

4. Joseph Herbert Kaufman, "Government Dentistry," *Dental Digest* 25 (November 1919): 647.

5. Ibid., 646–647.

6. T. P. Hyatt, "The Economic Value of the Industrial Dental Clinic," *Journal of the National Dental Association* 5 (October 1918): 1050–1052, and Thaddeus P. Hyatt, "Industrial Dentistry," *Dental Digest* 26 (April 1920): 248–249.

7. Weston A. Price, "The Responsibility of the Management for the Effect of Focal Infection (Especially Dental) on the Life, Health, and Efficiency of the Employee," *Dental Items of Interest* 47 (December 1925): 899.

8. Lee K. Frankel, "Dental Work in the Industries," *Dental Digest* 23 (July 1917): 452–457.

9. George J. Krakow, "Dental Inspection of Employees in Large Corporations," *The Dental Cosmos* 58 (December 1916): 1384.

10. Ibid., 1386.

11. Frankel, "Dental Work in the Industries," 454.

12. Louis P. Cardwell, "Industrial Dentistry," *Dental Digest* 26 (June 1920): 336.

13. Frankel, "Dental Work in the Industries," 455.

14. Arthur Williams, "Industry and the Health of the Employe," as reprinted in the *Journal of the National Dental Association* 5 (September 1918): 954.

15. As cited in Colin Gordon, *Dead on Arrival: The Politics of Health Care in Twentieth-Century America* (Princeton, NJ: Princeton University Press, 2003): 16.

16. For more detail on the development of health insurance plans in the 1920s and 1930s and the role of the AMA in that process, see Paul Starr, *The Social Transformation of American Medicine: The Rise of a Sovereign Profession and the Making of a Vast Industry* (New York: Basic Books, 1982), especially book 2, chapter 1, "The Mirage of Reform."

17. A. C. Wherry, "Dentistry's Duty to Humanity," *Dental Items of Interest* 55 (July 1933): 505.

18. Elizabeth Haiken, *Venus Envy: A History of Cosmetic Surgery* (Baltimore: Johns Hopkins University Press, 1997): 92. On the substitution of body modification for religious ritual, also see Joan Jacobs Brumberg, *Fasting Girls: The Emergence of Anorexia Nervosa as a Modern Disease* (Cambridge: Harvard University Press, 1988), and *The Body Project: An Intimate History of American Girls* (New York: Random House, 1997).

19. *Good Housekeeping* 40 (June 1930): 153.

20. Ibid.

21. *Betty's Crooked Teeth* (Producer unknown, circa 1937).

22. Editorial, "Pauperized by Health Service Not by Education," *Journal of the Michigan State Dental Society* 15 (February 1933): 25.

23. Ibid., 26.

24. Rubin Slater, "Medicine and Dentistry, as Education, Should Be Socialized," *Dental Outlook* 20 (September 1933): 391.

25. G. W. Haigh, "State Medicine: A Vanishing Bogey," *Dental Outlook* 20 (October 1933): 431.

26. Slater, "Medicine and Dentistry, as Education, Should Be Socialized," 393.

27. Haigh, "State Medicine," 435.

28. Ibid.

29. Slater, "Medicine and Dentistry, as Education, Should Be Socialized," 391.

30. James Howell, "Dentistry in Northern Russia," *Bulletin of the Michigan State Dental Society* 1 (March 1919): 5

31. "Bolshevism Due to Teeth, Says Dentist," *Oral Hygiene* 13 (May 1923): "Sepia Section," unpaginated.

32. "American Dentistry in Siberia," *Dental Digest* 25 (June 1919): 372.

33. Charles H. H. Ritter, "The American Plan to Guarantee Everybody Equal Opportunity to Enjoy the Blessings of Scientific Dentistry," *Journal of the American Dental Association* 20 (February 1933): 318.

34. I. A. Gershanski, "The Present State of Dentistry in Soviet Russia," *Journal of the American Dental Association* 16 (October 1929): 1871. Gershanski was a dentist who, by 1930, was serving as first assistant in the (Ukraine) Department of Social Odontology. (George Randorf, "Odontology and Stomatology in Soviet Russia for the Past Decade [fifth in a series]," *Dental Digest* 36 [December 1930]: 784.)

35. Gershanski, "The Present State of Dentistry in Soviet Russia," 1873.

36. Ibid.

37. Randorf," Odontology and Stomatology in Soviet Russia," 786.

38. Solomon Gross, "Health! Toward Economic Security," *The Dental Cosmos* 78 (August 1936): 875–876.

39. Interview with Peter Swanish, "Dentistry in Soviet Russia," *Dental Digest* 38 (January 1932): 27.

40. Edward Ochsner, "Social Insurance," *Northwest Journal of Dentistry* 21 (January 1933): 23.

41. "Socialized Medicine," *Bulletin of the National Dental Association* 8 (October 1949): 37–38. The journal of the National Dental Association was titled, variously, the *Bulletin of the National Dental Association*, the *Quarterly of the National Dental Association*, and the *NDA Journal*.

42. Ochsner, "Social Insurance," 23.

43. Douglas W. Stephens, "After We've Fought and Won," *Dental Items of Interest* 66 (February 1944): 159–160.

44. "A War Angle in Dental Health Teaching: Danville, Pennsylvania Public Schools," *The Journal of the American Dental Hygienists' Association* 18 (January 1944): 12.

45. Thomas L. Hagain, "Dentistry for Civilians in Wartime," *Journal of the American Dental Association* 31 (June 1944): 847, and Stephens, "After We've Fought and Won," 163.

46. Alfred J. Asgis, "*Inimical* to the Best Interests of the Public and the Science and Practice of Dentistry," *Texas Dental Journal* 61 (October 1943): 393. At his death, Asgis was described as a "dynamic adversary of lower-level dentistry" and an "opponent of commercialism." Joseph H. Kauffman, "Alfred J. Asgis, 1893–1979, Devoted Life to Dental Profession," *New York State Dental Journal* 45 (August/September 1979): 341.

47. Editorial, "Inimical," *Texas Dental Journal* 61 (August 1943): 303.

48. Charles Hardy, "Something to Think About," *Journal of the New Jersey State Dental Society* 15 (January 1944), 34.

49. Columbus Giragi, "Dental Licensing Versus Democracy," *Oral Hygiene* 38 (October 1948): 1561.

50. Editorial, "Wanted: Pioneers for Dentistry's Frontier, the Small Towns of America," *Dental Survey* 22 (September 1946): 1687.

51. Dean Howard, "The Aftermath" (Meharry Medical School Commencement Address of June 1943), as published by the *Meharri-Dent* 2 (December 1943): 32.

52. "Socialized Medicine," *Bulletin of the National Dental Association,* 37–38.

53. William R. Gubbins, "Let's Look Into This Unionism Business," *Oral Hygiene* 32 (January 1942): 43.

54. Howard, "The Aftermath," 32.

55. Alfred Asgis, "Postwar Dentistry: A Program," *Dental Items of Interest* 65 (May 1943): 467.

56. Alfred Asgis, "Quality Dentistry for American Labor," *Oral Hygiene* 35 (July 1945): 1193.

57. On AMA opposition to Wagner-Murray-Dingell and the Truman administration's health care plan, see Starr, *The Social Transformation of American Medicine,* especially pages 280–289.

58. Alfred Asgis, "American Labor Wants Dental Care," *Oral Hygiene* 34 (September 1944): 1459.

59. George Schneider, "A New Approach to Federal Dental Health Insurance," *Oral Hygiene* 39 (July 1949): 1068.

60. R. B. Moore, "Will Compulsory Health Insurance Fail?" *Dental Students' Magazine* 27 (June 1949): 26.

61. Kenneth A. Easlick, "Milestones: A Resume of Health Laws Passed and Proposed During the Past 40 Years," *Journal of the American Dental Association* 38 (April 1949): 484, 491.

62. Max Ernst, "President's Address, American Association of Orthodontists," as reprinted by the *American Journal of Orthodontics* 36 (November 1950): 809. The legislation was a drastically reduced version of Wagner-Murray-Dingell. Though some increases to a tightly circumscribed program of health insurance for the aged were passed in 1950, Medicare would not be created as a separate program until fifteen years later (Starr, *The Social Transformation of American Medicine,* 280–286).

63. On postwar health-care bargaining, see Gordon, *Dead on Arrival,*especially pages 60–67.

64. Henry Klein, "Civilian Dentistry in War-Time," *Journal of the American Dental Association* 31 (May 1944): 660. Wartime productivity guru W. Edwards Deming, then employed by the federal Bureau of the Budget, assisted in Klein's research.

Chapter 5 — Behind the Fluorine Curtain

1. The characteristic stain of fluorosis was also, much less frequently (and almost never after about 1925), referred to as "Naples stain," because a group of Italian immigrants from Pozzuoli, a community outside of Naples, had demonstrated signs of the condition as early as 1901 (Bureau of Public Relations, "Endemic Dental Fluorosis or Mottled Enamel," *Journal of the American Dental Association* 30 [August 1943]: 1278).

2. Frederick McKay, "Mottled Enamel: A Fundamental Problem in Dentistry," *The Dental Cosmos* 67 (September 1925): 848.

3. Ibid., 852.

4. Ibid.

5. Ibid.

6. Ibid.

7. Ibid., 855, 857.

8. "Endemic Dental Fluorosis or Mottled Enamel," *Journal of the American Dental Association,*1279.

9. The earliest federally funded dental research, as Ruth Roy Harris has pointed out, was spurred by widespread interest in the phenomenon of mottled enamel. Ruth Roy Harris, *Dental Science in a New Age: A History of the National Institute of Dental Research* (Rockville, MD: Montrose Press, 1989): 45–50.

10. Letter of C. T. Messner to Hugh Cumming, July 6, 1927, National Archives and Records Administration, RG 90 Records of the Public Health Service, Box 890, File 0412 General (1921–1934).

11. Viron Diefenbach et al., "Fluoridation and the Appearance of Teeth," *Journal of the American Dental Association* 71 (November 1965): 1129.

12. "Endemic Dental Fluorosis or Mottled Enamel," *Journal of the American Dental Association*,1282–1283.

13. Letter of H. Trendley Dean to Hugh Cumming, December 9, 1932, National Archives and Records Administration, RG 90 Records of the Public Health Service, Box 890, File 0412 General (1921–1934).

14. Gary Regenbaum, "The Water Fluoridation Controversy," *Dental Students' Magazine* 45 (October 1966): 88.

15. Paul Morgan, "Public Drinking Water May Fight Tooth Decay," *Dental Health* 1 (November 1942): 7.

16. Committee to Protect our Children's Teeth, *Our Children's Teeth: A Digest of Expert Opinion Based on Studies of the Use of Fluorides in Public Water Supplies* (New York: CPOCT, 1957): 21. This disagreement about what aesthetic changes counted as problems in need of resolution persisted. Contemplating the increase of the Environmental Protection Agency's "maximum allowable" fluoride level from two to four parts per million in 1985, US Surgeon General C. Everett Koop admitted that fluoride at such a concentration could cause aesthetic damage, but concluded that: "It's only cosmetic." Dorothy Link Donohoe and Thomas L. Donohoe, *Fluoride/Fluoridation: Understanding It, Updating, and Getting it Together Now*, 2nd ed. (Self-published, 1988): 93.

17. "Citizen Groups, Doctors Speak Out On Fluoridation," Week of December 12, 1962, Wayne State University Archives of Labor and Urban Affairs and University Archives, Cavanaugh collection, Box 82, Cavanaugh folder.

18. "Suburbs Seek to Cut City's Water Authority," *Detroit News*, March 8, 1963.

19. Speech of Maurice Reitzer, April 22, 1976, reprinted in Dental Division, Michigan Department of Public Health, *Fluoridation: Resource Guide for Speakers* (Lansing: Michigan DPH, 1981): C-6, C-2.

20. A. A. London, "Speaking Out," *National Fluoridation News* 11, no. 4 (July-August 1965): 3, as cited in Gretchen Reilly, "This Poisoning of Our Drinking Water" (Ph.D. dissertation, George Washington University, 2001).

21. Ohio Pure Water Association, "Facts about Fluoridation: Your Health and Your Human Rights Are at Stake," pamphlet, Wayne State University Archives of Labor and Urban Affairs and University Archives, Cavanaugh collection, Box 82, Folder 12.

22. Fanchon Battelle, *Fluoridation Unmasked* (Wisconsin, Royal Lee, 1953): 16.

23. Mary Berhnardt, "Fluoridation: How Far in 20 Years?" *Journal of the American Dental Association* 71 (November 1965): 1117. See also David Ast et al., "Time and Cost Factors to Provide Regular, Periodic Dental Care for Children in a Fluoridated and Nonfluoridated Area: Final Report," *Journal of the American Dental Association* 80 (April 1970): 770–778.

24. For "ghastly," see "Endemic Dental Fluorosis or Mottled Enamel," *Journal of the American Dental Association,* 1278. For reports of superoxol bleaching, see H. V. Smith and John W. McInnes, "Further Studies on Methods of Removing Brown Stain from Mottled Teeth," *Journal of the American Dental Association* 29 (April 1942): 575.

25. Harold B. Younger, "Bleaching Mottled Enamel," *Texas Dental Journal* 60 (December 1942): 469.

26. Medical-Dental Committee on Evaluation of Fluoridation, *Current Status of the Fluoridation Discussion,* 2nd ed. (Boonton, NJ: MCDEF, 1963): 33.

27. F. B. Exner, "Fluoride: A Protected Pollutant/Economic Motives behind Fluoridation," address to the Western Conference of Natural Food Associates, Salt Lake City, Utah, October 27, 1961, as reproduced at http://www.fluoridation.com/exner. htm, accessed July 13, 2000, emphasis in original.

28. "Two Views on Fluoridation," circa 1963, no publication information available, located in Wayne State University Archive of Labor and Urban Affairs and University Archive, Cavanaugh collection, Box 257, Folder 8.

29. For details, see Paul Starr, *The Social Transformation of American Medicine: The Rise of a Sovereign Profession and the Making of a Vast Industry* (New York: HarperCollins, 1982).

30. "Denies Sodium Fluoride is Industry's Waste Product," *Journal of the American Dental Association* 51 (September 1955): 373.

31. Richard Buck, "Fluoridation Education," *Dental Students' Magazine* 45 (November 1966): 140.

32. Leon R. Kramer, "A Challenge to High School Students," *Dental Health* 2 (February 1943): 2.

33. "Citizen Groups, Doctors Speak Out On Fluoridation," unidentified source recorded in handwriting as "Week of December 12, 1962," Wayne State University Archives of Labor and Urban Affairs and University Archives, Cavanaugh collection, Box 82, Cavanaugh folder.

34. Letter of James H. Lincoln to Jerome P. Cavanaugh, January 2, 1963, Wayne State University Archives of Labor and Urban Affairs and University Archives, Cavanaugh collection, Box 82, Folder 12. On racial tension in postwar Detroit, see Thomas Sugrue, *The Origins of the Urban Crisis: Race and Inequality in Postwar Detroit* (Princeton, NJ: Princeton University Press, 1996).

35. Letter of James H. Lincoln to Jerome P. Cavanaugh, January 2, 1963.

36. William Travis, "Fluoridation Travesty," undated news item cut from unidentified source, Wayne State University Archives of Labor and Urban Affairs and University Archives, Cavanaugh collection, Box 257, Folder 8.

37. Letter of Mrs. McRouth to Jerome P. Cavanaugh, February 13, 1962, Wayne State University Archives of Labor and Urban Affairs and University Archives, Cavanaugh collection, Box 25, Folder 2.

38. "Citizens of the City of Detroit, Wayne, Oakland and Macomb Counties: Unless You Act Promptly You Will Be Drinking Water With a Poison Chemical Whether You Like It Or Not!" Detroit Citizens Studying Fluoridation, circa 1965, Wayne State University Archives of Labor and Urban Affairs and University Archives, Cavanaugh collection, Box 25, Folder 21.

39. Ibid.

40. "The P.T.A. Council and the Board of Education distributed via the school children approximately 380,000 flyers alerting parents to beware" of the confusing

wording of the ballot question on fluoridation (which would have prohibited the fluoridation of public water supplies, meaning that a "no" vote was necessary to express a favorable attitude towards fluoride) in Detroit in 1965. Proponents of fluoridation won the referendum by about 6,000 votes. (William Travis, "Detroit Gains Fluoridation," *Journal of the Michigan State Dental Association* 47 [December 1965]: 355, and Martin Naimark, "Not to Be Denied," *Detroit Dental Bulletin* 34 [December 1965]: 6.)

41. Travis, "Detroit Gains Fluoridation," 361.

42. F. L. Losee, "Fluoride, Good or Bad?" *Journal of the American Dental Association* 69 (August 1964): 254. For more discussion of Social Security and Medicare, see Chapter 5, and Starr, *The Social Transformation of American Medicine*, especially pages 367–378, on "Redistributive Reform and Its Impact."

43. Ohio Pure Water Association, "Facts About Fluoridation: Your Health and Your Human Rights Are At Stake".

44. Letter of Mrs. Roy Percy to Mayor Jerome Cavanaugh, Wayne State University Archives of Labor and Urban Affairs and University Archives, Cavanaugh collection, Box 82, Folder 12.

45. "Fluoridation Wins in New York City," *Journal of the American Dental Association* 68 (January 1964): 105.

46. F. A. Bull, "Water Fluorination Proves Its Value," *Dental Digest* 55 (June 1949): 257.

47. W. Hume Everett, "Your Fraternity and Your American Heritage," *Texas Dental Journal* 81 (July 1963): 10, 11.

48. "Citizens of the City of Detroit, Wayne, Oakland and Macomb Counties." Detroit Citizens Studying Fluoridation. And, of course, anxiety about Detroit's failure to "respect city limits" reflected fears that the city's growing racial tension and resultant disorder would spill over into the Wayne, Oakland, and Macomb County suburbs where former white residents of the city had fled.

49. Undated letter of (Mrs.) Elma Ambrose to Jerome P. Cavanaugh, Wayne State University Archives of Labor and Urban Affairs and University Archives, Cavanaugh collection, Box 25, Folder 2.

50. "Citizens of the City of Detroit, Wayne, Oakland and Macomb Counties," Detroit Citizens Studying Fluoridation.

51. "Suburbs Seek to Cut City's Water Authority," *Detroit News*, March 8, 1963.

52. J. E. Waters in *Dental Survey* 29 (November 1953), as cited in William McGrath, "The Fallacy of Fluoridation," (Scarboro Missions pamphlet circa 1956), located in Wayne State University Archives of Labor and Urban Affairs and University Archives, Cavanaugh collection, Box 25, Folder 20.

53. Fanchon Battelle, *Fluoridation Unmasked* (Wisconsin: Royal Lee, 1953): 5, 7. The specificity of Battelle's fears, and their failure of fruition, makes them seem ludicrous in retrospect. The general suspicion that the US government might contemplate the use of chemicals for mind control was not: the Central Intelligence Agency was then undertaking experiments with lysergic acid dimethylamine (LSD) in an attempt to find a "truth serum" that could be used on Communist informants. (See Martin Lee, *Acid Dreams: The CIA, LSD and the Sixties Rebellion* [New York: Grove Press, 1985].)

54. Historical, sociological, and political science studies examining the bases of opposition to water fluoridation constituted something of a cottage industry in

the 1960s and 1970s (though, perversely, relatively few researchers ever set out to determine why someone might approve of water fluoridation). Two examples of studies that include the consideration of both positions are: John E. Mueller, "The Politics of Fluoridation in Seven California Cities," *The Western Political Quarterly* 19 (March 1966): 54–67, and A. Stafford Metz, "The Relationship of Dental Care Practices to Attitude toward Fluoridation," *Journal of Health and Social Behavior* 8 (March 1967): 55–59.

55. In 1970, John Knutson reported that "the antifluoridationists won in almost two thirds of the approximately 900 public referendums held in communities to determine the fate of water fluoridation" between 1955 and 1965. John Knutson, "Water Fluoridation after 25 Years," *Journal of the American Dental Association* 80 (April 1970): 767.

56. The claim was rendered completely in capitalized type. "Citizens of the City of Detroit, Wayne, Oakland and Macomb Counties," Detroit Citizens Studying Fluoridation.

57. Randolph Bishop, "What Can the Public Expect of Fluorine?" *Dental Health* (August, 1945): 11. The occurrence of ills attributed by an anxious public to the effects of fluoridated water was frequently cited, always with amusement, by pro-fluoridationists. "Almost traditional in fluoridation," remarked Mary Bernhardt in the *Journal of the American Dental Association* in 1965, "are the imaginary ailments that afflict persons in a community before the fluoride has been put in the water. Complaints range from nausea to bad-tasting coffee. Even the deaths of goldfish have been blamed on fluoridation." [Bernhardt, "Fluoridation: How Far in 20 Years?" 1120.]

58. Bureau of Public Information, "Comments on the Opponents of Fluoridation," *Journal of the American Dental Association* 71 (November 1965): 1172–1173. The list of fluoridation opponents in the article was quite comprehensive, including both individuals and organizations, and catalogued objections to fluoridation raised by everyone down to the John Birch Society and the Ku Klux Klan, whose presence on the list seems to have been intended to tar everyone else by association (as the Klan was not, as even the article itself admitted, a particularly potent antifluoridation force).

59. William Travis, "What Do They Say?" *Detroit Dental Bulletin* 34 (April 1965): 8.

60. William Travis, "Who Are They?" *Detroit Dental Bulletin* 34 (January 1965): 11.

61. Knutson, "Water Fluoridation after 25 Years," 766, and William Wickers, "The Affirmative Case for Fluoridation," *Journal of the Tennessee State Dental Association* 43 (July 1963): 221. The derisive use of the term "professional" to describe anti-fluoridation activists suggests how firmly the word had become associated with high educational and social status: antfluoridationists could be mockingly described as "professional" precisely because they were understood by dentists to lack hard-earned "professional" qualities, and the good judgment that came with them.

62. Bernhardt, "Fluoridation—How Far in 20 Years?" 1117.

63. As David Chappell has demonstrated, quiet white Southern support for the civil rights movement was critical to the movement's success, and the influence of white and black "outside agitators," though bitterly resented by segregationists, has been overestimated. At the time, however, the currency of the reference was extremely powerful. See David Chappell, *Inside Agitators: White*

Southerners in the Civil Rights Movement (Baltimore: Johns Hopkins University Press, 1994).

64. William Travis, "Whom Do You Believe?" *Journal of the Michigan State Dental Association* 48 (April 1966): 182.

65. Maynard K. Hine, "Address by Dr. Maynard K. Hine, President, ADA," *Oregon State Dental Journal* 35 (June 1966): 9.

66. Emma Carr Bivins, "People Are Giving Us the Answers," *Journal of the American Dental Association* 71 (November 1965): 1151.

67. On feminist opposition to medical authority, see The Boston Women's Health Book Collective, *Our Bodies, Ourselves: A Book By and For Women* (New York: Simon and Schuster, 1971).

68. Hine, "Address by Dr. Maynard K. Hine, President, ADA," 9.

69. Travis, "Whom Do You Believe?" 182.

70. H. William Gross, "How To Take the Controversy Out of Fluoridation," *Pennsylvania Dental Journal* 31 (May 1964): 144.

71. William Travis, "Why Not Fluoridate Milk?" *Detroit Dental Bulletin* 31 (July 1962): 6, emphasis in original.

72. Bivins, "People Are Giving Us the Answers," 1151.

73. "Trenton—The All-America Fluoridated City," *Journal of the New Jersey State Dental Society* 38 (September 1966): 28–29.

74. "'Flora Who?'" *Dental Students' Magazine* 47 (November 1968): 140.

75. "News of Dentistry," *Journal of the American Dental Association* 71 (November 1965): 1203.

Chapter 6 — The "Satisfaction of Dentistry" and the End of Public Health

1. J. A. Salzmann and David B. Ast, "The Newburgh-Kingston Fluorine Study, IX: Dentofacial Growth and Development—Cephalometric Study," *American Journal of Orthodontics* 41 (1955): 674, as cited in J. A. Salzmann, "Fluoridation and Changes in Orthodontic Practice," *American Journal of Orthodontics* 52 (October 1966): 780.

2. Nelson Cruikshank, "Labor Looks at Dental Prepayment," *Journal of the American Dental Association* 69 (August 1964): 88.

3. Colin Gordon, *Dead on Arrival: The Politics of Health Care in Twentieth-Century America* (Princeton, NJ: Princeton University Press, 2003): 30.

4. See Lizabeth Cohen, *A Consumer's Republic: The Politics of Mass Consumption in America* (New York: Knopf, 2003), especially pages 408 and 409: "Increasingly over this century, the economic behavior of consumption has become entwined with the rights and obligations of citizenship. . . . In America . . . it was the private consumer economy—not a welfare state, though on many occasions government assisted—that was charged with the responsibility of fulfilling the nation's economic obligations to its citizens."

5. *Mindblower: Dental Profession under Siege* (Produced by the American Dental Association, 1978). The film, which was under four minutes in length, consisted of a rapidly changing montage of newspaper and magazine headlines trumpeting public anger about the high cost and low quality of health care. The musical accompaniment was "Dueling Banjos," a song already well-known to Americans for its role in the soundtrack of the 1972 film *Deliverance*, in which the competitive

playing of the song served as a harbinger of the conflicts between civilization and savagery that would occur later in the movie.

6. Robert Stinaff, "Effect of Dental Hygienists and Dental Assistants on the Production of Dental Care," *Journal of the American Dental Association* 60 (January 1960): 54.

7. George Ward Glann, "Effect of Dental Hygienists and Dental Assistants on the Economics and Management of the Dental Practice," *Journal of the American Dental Association* 60 (January 1960): 61.

8. Albert Peyraud, "Glamour for the Dental Assistant," *CAL* 30 (July 1967): 8–10. A year earlier, in his address to the Wisconsin Dental Study Club, Peyraud listed "femininity" first, "education" fourth, and "good appearance" eleventh. (Albert Peyraud, address to the Wisconsin Dental Study Club, August 17, 1966, as published by *CAL* 29 (October 1966): 23–24.

9. Peyraud, "Glamour for the Dental Assistant," 7.

10. George Crane, "Are You Guilty of Psychological Malpractice?" *CAL* 25 (February 1963): 17.

11. Betty Gray, "The Other Women in Your Husband's Life!" *CAL* 30 (July 1967): 20. Gray authored a running column for dental wives that included advice on how women could positively affect their husbands' attitudes (and, thereby, their productivity at work and the success of their practices): one such column advised wives to "show your affection and intelligence by looking kissable and cheerful in your breakfast attire. If there are children to consider, keep them orderly and agreeable. Avoid arguments and dissensions. It is your duty, dear wife, to see to it that the family breakfast is pleasant as well as nourishing." (Betty Gray, "The Happy Home," *CAL* 30 [November 1967]: 10.)

12. One exception came in 1979, in "Your Aide vs. 'The Octopus': How to Fend off Unwanted Advances without Offending Patients," which was addressed to dentists, not their assistants. (*Dental Management* 19 [January 1979]: 22–24.)

13. Cartoon, *CAL* 30 [July 1967]: 11.

14. "The Case of Fran and the Beautician's Pay," *CAL* 29 (January 1967): 21.

15. Ibid.

16. "Who Deserves More? Beautician or D.A.?" *CAL* 29 (May 1967): 1.

17. Ibid.

18. For examples that bracketed a forty-year span: "Previous experience in another dental office is considered a disadvantage rather than an advantage" (C. Edmund Kells, *The Dentist's Own Book* [St. Louis: C. V. Mosby Company, 1925]: 290). And: "If you hire a person with previous dental office experience, you may be unhappy with her" (Harold J. Ashe, "Search for These Traits in an Assistant," *Oral Hygiene* 55 [October 1965]: 49).

19. On teachers, for example, see Marjorie Murphy, *Blackboard Unions: The AFT and the NEA, 1900–1980* (Ithaca, NY: Cornell University Press, 1990), especially page 209: "By the late seventies, 72 percent of all public school teachers were members of some form of union that represented them at the bargaining table. Before 1961 unions in less than a dozen school districts could claim they represented only a small fraction of teachers." On clerical workers, see John Hoerr, *We Can't Eat Prestige: The Women Who Organized Harvard* (Philadelphia: Temple University Press, 1997).

20. Cyril Kanterman, "De-Sexing the Dental Office," *Dental Students' Magazine* 44 (December 1965): 223. Kanter, drawing on the extreme example of the "Playboy bunny" to demonstrate that not all jobs ought to be open to all people, predicted that "dentistry's bunny problem may or may not be solved to everyone's full satisfaction. We doubt if anybody's bunny problem will be of easy solution" (223).

21. John C. Cushman, "Relations between Dentistry and Organized Labor—Do's and Don'ts in Labor Relations," as published by the *Journal of the Southern California State Dental Association* 33 (July 1965): 293.

22. Keith Sutherland, "Your Employees Need Planning—*Not* Unionization," *Oral Hygiene* 57 (May 1967): 59.

23. "Anonymous," "A Disgruntled Employee Took Me to Labor Court," *Dental Economics* 67 (April 1977): 91–100. "As a dentist," he wrote, "the job of being an employer has potential risks as threatening as negligence at the chair in the operatory. The employee you hire could take you to court faster than any patient you will ever see" (100).

24. "Miscellaneous," *Bulletin of the National Dental Association* 12 (April 1954): 99.

25. "Great Expectations?" *Bulletin of the National Dental Association* 12 (January 1954): 60.

26. Ibid.

27. On affirmative action, see Harvey Webb, "Problems and Progress of Black Dental Professionals," *Quarterly of the National Dental Association* 34 (July 1976): 148. On Medicare, Medicaid, and federal educational aid, see James C. Wallace, "The National Dental Association and Its Contribution to American Dentistry," *Quarterly of the National Dental Association* 24 (January 1966): 44.

28. Texas Health Council, "Social Security: Facts and Fantasy," *Texas Dental Journal* 80 (December 1962): 17.

29. Lloyd French, "Dentists and Social Security," *Bulletin of the National Dental Association* 16 (July 1958): 99.

30. "Editorial: For the Health Professions, A Legacy," *Quarterly of the National Dental Association* 26 (July 1968): 89.

31. "1970 NDA Annual Meeting," *Quarterly of the National Dental Association* 29 (October 1970): 15.

32. Ibid.

33. John Conyers, "Black Political Strategy for 1972," *Quarterly of the National Dental Association* 30 (January 1972): 35.

34. Clifton O. Dummett, "Editorial: Professional Irresponsibility," *Quarterly of the National Dental Association* 30 (October 1971): 5.

35. See, for instance, Darlene Clark Hine's characterization of black nurses as "more so than any other black health-care professional, [bearing] the bulk of the responsibility to provide health-care services for, and to lift up from the bottom of the American social scale, the entire black race." (Darlene Clark Hine, *Black Women in White: Racial Conflict and Cooperation in the Nursing Profession 1890–1950* [Bloomington: Indiana University Press, 1989]: xvii.)

36. Caption, "Association News," *Quarterly of the National Dental Association* 36 (October 1977): 25.

37. Caption, "Association News," *Quarterly of the National Dental Association* 36 (April 1978): 97. The women in question may have been cast members of

Bubbling Brown Sugar, a musical portraying Harlem's golden years that opened on Broadway in 1976, but the caption did not identify the women as actresses, and its wording seemed calculated to invoke the popular understanding of "bubbling brown sugar" as a descriptor of black women's sexual charm—or, indeed, of their genitalia proper.

38. "She Tries to Raise "Dental IQ" in Black People," *Ebony* 33 (August 1978): 138.

39. Ibid., 139.

40. "Dental Dean," *Ebony* 28 (March 1973): 85.

41. Ibid., 85, 88, 90.

42. As late as 1976, Harvey Webb reported that "Despite [the ADA's 1961 nondiscrimination directive]. . . . vestiges of racial discrimination still persist in chapters [of the ADA] in many areas throughout the country. Some constituencies have never accepted a Black dentist to their membership." (Webb, "Problems and Progress of Black Dental Professionals," 152.)

43. "The Color Guard," *Journal of the American Dental Association* 68 (June 1964): 136.

44. Richard Basch, Letter to the Editor, "On 'The Color Guard,'" *Journal of the American Dental Association* 69 (August 1964): 162.

45. James Webb, Letter to the Editor, "A Reader Objects," *Journal of the American Dental Association* 69 (August 1964): 162.

46. Roger Spencer, Letter to the Editor, "Intolerance," *Journal of the American Dental Association* 69 (September 1964): 132.

47. Interview with Reginald Hawkins, "The Way the Color Line Cuts in Dentistry," *Dental Management* 5 (July 1965): 41.

48. Ibid., 46.

49. Editorial, "Negro Membership," *Journal of the American Dental Association* 71 (August 1965): no page number.

50. Ibid. Of course, many of the black dentists who might have applied for membership in the ADA were, by virtue of their involvement in the NDA, already "active members of organized dentistry."

51. William Garrett, "Intraprofessional Cooperation," *Quarterly of the National Dental Association* 25 (October 1966): 5–6.

52. Joseph L. Henry, "Where Do We Go from Here?" as published by the *Quarterly of the National Dental Association* 26 (October 1967): 6.

53. Joseph Henry used this term to differentiate the one third of black dentists who were paying members of the NDA—and who received its journal as part of their membership subscriptions—from a larger imagined population of those who merely sympathized with the organization's aims. Henry, "Where Do We Go from Here?" 5.

54. Robert Eilers, "An Independent National Agency for Dental Service Corporations?" *Journal of the American Dental Association* 69 (August 1964): 79.

55. Joseph Yany Bloom, "I Resigned from the Group Health Dental Insurance Program," *The Journal of the New Jersey State Dental Society* 34 (September 1962): 17.

56. Ramon Tappero, "Till All Liberty Shall Be Lost," *Journal of the California Dental Association* 441 (February 1965): 23.

57. Wayne Speer, "The Dental Service Corporation," *Texas Dental Journal* 80 (November 1962): 19.

58. Arthur Takamoto, Letter to the Editor, "National Association of Dental Service Plans," *Journal of the California Dental Association* 41 (February 1965): 32–33.

59. George Crane, "Are You Guilty of Psychological Malpractice? Adopt Four Sets of 'Twins' to Strengthen the Bulwark of Your Private Dental Practice," *CAL* 25 (February 1963): 17–18.

60. Jean Waller, "Cause and Cure of the Cash Register Complex," *Dental Management* 8 (December 1968): 38–41.

61. Ibid., 43.

62. H. Barry Waldman, "Must 8 specialties = 7 specialists + 1 traitor?" *New York Journal of Dentistry* 43 (December 1973): 315.

63. Walter Wilson, "The Future Role of Government in Dental Practice and Education," *Journal of the American College of Dentistry* 40 (April 1973): 111–116, as cited by Robert Wollman, "Current Socio-Economic and Political Changes and Their Effects on the Future Practice of Dentistry," *Illinois Dental Journal* 45 (November 1976): 561.

64. Wilson R. Flint, "President's Address," as published by the *American Journal of Orthodontics* 36 (March 1950): 166.

65. Wollman, "Current Socio-economic and Political Changes and Their Effects," 561.

66. Wayne Speer, "The Dental Service Corporation," *Texas Dental Journal* 80 (November 1962): 19.

67. Waller, "Cause and Cure of the Cash Register Complex," 38.

Chapter 7 — The Look of the American Mouth

1. See, for example, Sidney Kohn, "Pedodontic Progress and Cultural Advancement," *Journal of the New Jersey State Dental Society* 33 (January 1962): especially page 182, where Kohn argues "Careful attention to the dental needs of tomorrow's adults implies a cultural awareness on the part of a progressive profession. . . . it becomes incumbent upon us, if we are to maintain our autonomy and rights of self determination as a profession, to make the wisest and best possible use of our present resources in manpower, knowledge and abilities." Also, John Abel, "Socioeconomic Trends Relating to Orthodontics," as published by the *American Journal of Orthodontics* 48 (December 1962): 893–899.

2. Edward Podolsky, "Teeth and Behavior in Children," *Dental Items of Interest* 70 (October 1948): 1051.

3. J. A. Salzmann, "Orthodontics as a Public Health Activity," *American Journal of Orthodontics* 35 (March 1949): 180.

4. "Orthodontics: Questions and Answers," as published by the *American Journal of Orthodontics* 36 (August 1950): 621.

5. Clair Picard, "Surgical Correction of Mandibular Prognathism," *Dental Survey* 40 (March 1964): 35. To the best of my knowledge, I am unrelated to this author.

6. Harold Born, "Aids in Case Presentation," as published by the *American Journal of Orthodontics* 46 (February 1960): 110. Born recommended that orthodontists try to find at least one of the child patient's facial features to compliment. "When you really get hard up with respect to finding some nice feature to mention, other than to say that the patient has two eyes or a head, you can always find a feature that is simliar [sic] to either the father or the mother and mention it. This does not

necessarily mean that you like the feature, but you can rest assured that it will not displease the parent you are referring to" (111).

7. Ibid., 111.

8. Henry Lerian, "Facial Esthetics in Orthodontic Treatment," *International Journal of Orthodontics* 6 (December 1968): 99.

9. Neil Sushner, "A Photography Study of the Soft-Tissue Profile of the Negro Population," *American Journal of Orthodontics* 72 (October 1977): 373.

10. For example, see interview with Charles Post, "Art, Children, Dentistry: A Satisfying Combination," *Dental Student* 52 (December 1973): 48. "There's something artistic about dentistry," said Post, an orthodontist, "and that ties in with my natural proclivity towards art."

11. Personal communication to the author.

12. "A cheerful greeting should be extended to the child and the parent, and the youngster is greeted by his first name." Jacob Stolzenberg, "Suggestion: An Adjunct in Orthodontic Treatment," *American Journal of Orthodontics* 36 (March 1950): 201.

13. In the 1950s and 1960s, a large body of writing formed around the intersection of dentistry and psychoanalytic theory. In this analysis, work in the mouth threatened the child's most primal means of obtaining pleasure, and children's fears of the dentist were caused by imagined psychosexual threats rather than by genuine fears of pain. Theorists who held this view considered it especially important to keep parents out of sight when children were receiving treatment. For example, see Sanford Lewis, "Psychosomatic Formulations in Dentistry," *Journal of the American Dental Association* 63 (November 1961): 626–632.

14. R. S. Callender et al., "Orthodontic Feedback," *Journal of Clinical Orthodontics* 10 (August 1976): 597.

15. George Anderson, "Years of Change," as published by the *American Journal of Orthodontics* 50 (July 1964): 526.

16. For orthodontists' affluence, see the address of University of North Carolina School of Dentistry Dean James Bawden, "An Outsider Looks at Orthodontics," as published by the *American Journal of Orthodontics* 53 (November 1967): 858–859. "In looking at the specialty of orthodontics," Bawden said, "I see a proud tradition of men who have enjoyed a high degree of success, not only in the treatment of their patients but also in terms of personal affluence and status. In fact, statistics show them to have been the most affluent of all the dental specialists."

17. Charles Fitz-Patrick, "Is Dental Appearance Important in Business?" *Oral Hygiene* 53 (August 1963): 53–54.

18. Anderson, "Years of Change," 525.

19. Ian Story, "Psychological Issues in Orthodontic Practice," *American Journal of Orthodontics* 52 (August 1966): 597.

20. "Thus, Negroes are more than 500 percent worse off in the dentist:population ratio than the total population generally." Joseph Henry, "Where Do We Go from Here?" as published by the *Quarterly of the National Dental Association* 26 (October 1967): 7. According to figures provided by the NDA and ADA, in 2007, there was approximately one NDA member dentist per 5,000 black Americans, and two dentists per 5,000 persons in the American population as a whole.

21. US Congress, Office of Technology Assessment, "Children's Dental Services under the Medicaid Program—Background Paper," OTA-BP-H-78 (Washington, DC: US Government Printing Office, October 1990): 2–3.
22. Ibid., 1.
23. T.J.S. Ginwalla et al., "Surgical Removal of Gingival Pigmentation," *Journal of the Indian Dental Association* 38 (June 1966): 147–150, in Clifton Dummett, "Psychogenic Concomitants of Oro-Mucosal Melano-Pigmentation," *Quarterly of the National Dental Association* 27 (October 1968): 14.
24. Dummett, "Psychogenic Concomitants of Oro-Mucosal Melano-Pigmentation," 17.
25. Ibid.
26. Advertisement: "Take a Good Look at Natural Coe-Lor," *Quarterly of the National Dental Association* 29 (April 1971): front advertising section.
27. Advertisement: "The Look is Natural When the Denture Base is Natural Coe-Lor," *Quarterly of the National Dental Association* 31 (October 1972): front advertising section.
28. Advertisement: "New Caulk Hy-Pro Lucitone Fibered Dark," *Quarterly of the National Dental Association* 32 (April 1974): advertising section.
29. Advertisement: "Are Bioblend Teeth Just for Patients Who Wear Mink?" *Quarterly of the National Dental Association* 26 (October 1967): back cover.
30. "Protection in Depth," *Ebony* 16 (November 1960): 5.
31. "No One Wants to Go Round with Me," *Ebony* 16 (December 1960): 7.
32. "Brush My Teeth after Every Meal?" *Ebony* 16 (January 1961): 29, and "Gleem," *Ebony* 16 (February 1961): 29.
33. "Your Dentist . . ." *Ebony* 27 (April 1972): 9.
34. "Strictly for Laughs," *Ebony* 30 (March 1975): 123.
35. "Strictly for Laughs," *Ebony* 31 (July 1976): 64.
36. There is also a long history of religious interest in spontaneous tooth adornment. Reformation Christians hailed gold teeth that appeared without the ministrations of a dentist as signs of divine intervention. And in the late twentieth century, a group of (mostly white) charismatic Christians in Toronto seized upon the appearance of gold dental work in the mouths of some 300 of its members as evidence of God's special favor on both its pastor and those blessed by dental transformation. Citing Psalm 81, verse 10 ("Open your mouth, and I will fill it"), Toronto Airport Christian Fellowship Pastor John Arnott told a reporter from *Christianity Today* that "this is a miracle that you don't have to be sick to get. Almost every person could use a little dental work of one kind or another." (James A. Beverley, "Dental Miracle Reports Draw Criticism," *Christianity Today* 43, May 24, 1999, 17.) Arnott allowed that some people had even been blessed with dental gold while watching videos of the revival, which were on sale in the church's gift shop. (CN$19.99) ("Go For the Gold," Toronto Airport Christian Fellowship, 1999.)
37. Hettie Jones, *Big Star Fallin' Mama: Five Women in Black Music* (New York: Viking Press, 1974): 38.
38. See, for example, Angela Y. Davis, *Blues Legacies and Black Feminism: Gertrude 'Ma' Rainey, Bessie Smith, and Billie Holiday* (New York: Pantheon Books, 1998).
39. Alan Lomax, *Mister Jelly Roll: The Fortunes of Jelly Roll Morton, New Orleans Creole and the "Inventor of Jazz"* (New York: Grove Press, 1950): 154.
40. Ibid., 155.

41. William Eric Perkins, "The Rap Attack: An Introduction," in Perkins, ed., *Droppin' Science: Critical Essays on Rap Music and Hip Hop Culture* (Philadelphia: Temple University Press, 1996): 2.

42. Tricia Rose, *Black Noise: Rap Music and Black Culture in Contemporary America* (Middletown, CT: Wesleyan University Press, 1994): especially pages 36–38.

43. November 8, 2002, as heard on 91.7 FM WUOM.

44. "Grillz," by D. Carter, C. Gipp, G. Hamler, C. Harris, R. Harrison, C. Haynes, A. Jones, B. Knowles, J. Mauldin, J. Phillps, P. Slayton, and T. Williams. Copyright © 2005 by 2 Kingpins Publishing, Air Control Music, Basajamba Music, Beyonce Publishing, EMI April Music Inc., Hitco South, Jackie Frost Music Inc., Paul Wall Publishing, Sam Swap Publishing, Shaniah Cymone Music, Sony/ATV Tunes LLC, TMWilliams Publishing, Universal Music Corporation, Universal Music–MGB Studios, and WB Music Corp.

45. Andrew Guy Jr., "Gold in the Mouth, but None in the Pocket: Employers Turned Off by Youth Fad," *Raleigh News and Observer*, October 27, 2002, page E1.

46. "That Golden Smile Likely a Drawback," *Houston Chronicle*, June 15, 2001, 1.

47. Ibid.

48. "The Truth about Teeth: Gold Caps May Look Cool, But They Hide Real Trouble," *Newsday*, August 5, 1992, 25.

49. Ibid.

50. "Bill to Take Bite Out of Dental Fad," *New Orleans Times-Picayune*, February 2, 1995, B4.

51. "Many Metro Teens Seek a 24K Smile: Gold Caps Popular, But Dentists Warn of Health Concerns," *Atlanta Journal and Constitution*, A1.

52. "Gold Teeth and School Decay," *Baltimore Sun*, December 20, 1994, 22A.

53. Ibid.

54. "Word of Mouth Helps 'Rapper Dentist Daddy' Corner Flashy Market," *Wall Street Journal*, July 19, 2001, A1, A4.

55. Ibid.

56. Ibid.

57. "Naturally, All Our Kids Wear Braces," *Wall Street Journal*, October 27, 1999: A4. The ad recalled the dental journal article in which one orthodontist advised others to "subtly point out that the good results of professional care as seen by friends, coworkers and employers are as much a status symbol as the big car in the driveway." (Fitz-Patrick, "Is Dental Appearance Important in Business?" 53–54.)

Epilogue

1. "Brits Resort to Pulling Own Teeth," http://edition.cnn.com/2007/WORLD/europe/10/15/england.dentists, accessed October 15, 2007.

2. "Loose Talk," *US Weekly* 692 (May 19, 1008): 22.

3. Claudia Kalb, "Move Over, Mona Lisa," *Newsweek*, December 14, 1998, 94.

4. Karen Springen, "Million Dollar Smile," *Newsweek*, March 7, 2005, 59.

5. Hilary and Piers DuPre, *A Genius in the Family* (New York: Vintage Press, 1998).

6. Elizabeth Hayt, "Blinding Them with Smiles," *New York Times*, September 18, 2000.

7. www.blondebutbright.blogspot.com/2004_07_20_archive.html.

8. "US Dentists Can't Make Nation's Teeth Any Damn Whiter," *The Onion* 39 (No. 15), April 23, 2003.

9. "Bizarro," as published by the *Ann Arbor News*, October 27, 2007.

10. "Last Exit to Springfield," original air date March 11, 1993.

11. Christopher Hitchens, "On the Limits of Self-Improvement, Part II," *Vanity Fair* (December 2007): 174–175.

12. Ian Urbina, "In Kentucky's Teeth, Toll of Poverty and Neglect," *New York Times*, December 24, 2007, accessed on www.nytimes.com.

13. Natalie Angier, "Roots and All: A History of Teeth," *New York Times*, August 5, 2003.

14. "Readers' Poll," *Best Life* (May 2008): 18.

15. As Elizabeth Haiken writes: "We have encouraged the belief that the only practical solution is the individual one. Our increasing tendency to individualize social problems of inequality suggests just how fundamentally we have lost faith in the possibility that commitment and collective action can transform the society in which we live." Elizabeth Haiken, *Venus Envy: A History of Cosmetic Surgery* (Baltimore: Johns Hopkins University Press, 1997): 15.

16. Mary Otto, "For Want of a Dentist: Prince George's Boy Dies after Bacteria from Tooth Spread to Brain," *Washington Post*, February 28, 2007.

17. Alex Berenson, "Boom Times for Dentists, But Not for Teeth," *New York Times*, October 11, 2007.

18. Otto, "For Want of a Dentist."

19. Berenson, "Boom Times for Dentists."

20. Ibid.

21. Steven Lauridsen, "Time for 'No Teeth Left Behind'?" Letters, *New York Times*, October 15, 2007.

Index

1918–1919 influenza pandemic, 38

acid reflux. *See* dyspepsia
activism, 8, 42, 134–138, 141–142, 176; of
   black dentists, 147–148, 152; and collective action, 152–153
advertising, 4, 9–10, 23, 32, 85, 87, 97–98,
   175, 186n32
Africa, 77, 80, 81, 82, 83, 85
African Americans, 6–7, 44–45, 111, 113,
   146–152, 163–174, 180
agriculture, 59–60, 69–70
alcohol, 46, 133, 197n36
Alinsky, Saul, 192n35
Allied Expeditionary Forces, 38
Aluminum Corporation of America, 121
American Academy of Cosmetic Dentistry,
   2
American Academy of Dental Science, 46
American Association for Labor Legislation, 100
American Association of Orthodontists,
   115
American Dental Assistants' Association,
   36, 67, 188n76
American Dental Association, 4, 7, 9, 10,
   52, 63, 66, 146, 147, 159, 176, 184; and
   dental insurance, 100, 105, 114, 143, 147,
   154; and fluoride, 122–123, 136, 139;
   racial segregation of, 142, 146, 150–152
American dentistry, 72–74, 77–80, 141; and
   business practices, 3, 9, 81–83, 98; and
   colonialism, 88–92, 98; international
   acclaim of, 77–78, 84–87, 175–178; and
   social status of dentists, 84
American Federation of Teachers, xi–xii,
   209n19
American Home Economics Association,
   50
American Idol (TV show), 175
Americanization: of immigrants, 14–15, 17,
   22–23, 27, 34–35, 37–38, 50, 61–62, 178

(*see also* assimilation of immigrants); of
   Native Hawai'ians, 94–98
American Medical Association, 5–6, 100,
   105, 108, 147, 201n16
Americans: attitudes toward work, 91–92,
   110–111; dental health habits of, 14, 19,
   39–41, 111–112, 128–129; genetic heritage of, 44, 47–48, 65; poor dental health
   of, 2, 41–42, 48, 54, 79, 98; reputation for
   good dental health of, 2, 39–41, 175–178
American Samoa, 67, 76
American social and economic systems,
   70, 128–129, 156, 168, 170, 172–174,
   208n4
anesthesia, 3, 4, 144, 197n36
Angier, Natalie, 179
Ann Arbor (Mich.), 162
anti-Communism. *See* Communism
anti-Semitism. *See* Jews
antisepsis, 3, 80
appearance, 2, 9, 14, 25–27, 74, 87, 89, 91,
   106–107, 118, 120–126, 158–174; and
   race, 161–174; and self-worth, 18–19,
   106–107, 125, 159–160, 178–179
appetite, 59–64
apprenticeship, 5–7, 43, 80
Armour & Co., 102, 104
Asgis, Alfred, 112, 114, 115, 202n46
Asians. *See* Chinese; Filipinos; Indians,
   Asian; Japanese
assimilation of immigrants, 11, 18, 191–
   192n34, 192n35. *See also* Americanization
assistants, dental. *See* dental assistants
Ast, David, 123
atavism. *See* degeneracy
Atlanta Journal and Constitution (newspaper), 171
Austin Powers (film series), 177–178
Australia, 68, 85

baby boom, 131, 143, 159
bacteriology, 3, 24, 49, 80

About the Author

Alyssa Picard is a graduate of the University of Michigan, where she received a PhD in history. She works as a negotiator for the American Federation of Teachers' Michigan state affiliate, and as an instructor in the history of social movements at Wayne State University's Labor School in Detroit.

Printed in the USA
CPSIA information can be obtained
at www.ICGtesting.com
LVHW020602041223
765568LV00002B/196